13.

under which I could accept the appointment. His knowledge of these conditions will aid you and your Committee in the discussion of the details which you mention in your letter as being necessary for consideration before the final appointment is offered me.

If I receive the appointment I should like to begin my work about the middle of May. i.e. before the present session ends.

With best wishes I am

Sincerely your

Duncan Graham

CANADIAN MEDICAL LIVES NO. 1

Duncan Graham

Medical Reformer and Educator

by
Robert B. Kerr, M.D.
and Douglas Waugh, M.D.

Series Editor: T.P. Morley, M.D.

Hannah Institute
&
Dundurn Press
Toronto and Oxford
1989

Design: Andy Tong
Printing and Binding: Gagné Printing Ltd., Louiseville, Quebec, Canada

Care has been taken to trace the ownership of copyright material used in the text (including the illustrations). The author and publisher welcome any information enabling them to rectify any reference or credit in subsequent editions.

J. Kirk Howard, Publisher

Canadian Cataloguing in Publication Data

Kerr, Robert B., 1908-
  Duncan Graham

(The Canadian Medical lives series ; 1)
Co-published by the Hannah Institute for the
History of Medicine
Includes bibliographical references and index.
ISBN 1-55002-046-3

1. Graham, Duncan, 1882-1974. 2. Physicians — Ontario — Biography. 3. University of Toronto. Faculty of Medicine — Faculty — Biography. 4. Medical teaching personnel — Ontario — Toronto — Biography. I. Waugh, Douglas, 1918-   . II. Hannah Institute for the History of Medicine. III. Title. IV. Series.

R464.G73K47 1988   610'.92'4   C89-093087-2

Dundurn Press Limited
2181 Queen Street East, Suite 301
Toronto, Canada
M4E 1E5

Dundurn Distribution Limited
Athol Brose, School Hill,
Wargrave, Reading
England
RG10 8DY

Canadian Medical Lives Series

The story of the Hannah Institute for the History of Medicine has been told by John B. Neilson and G.R. Paterson in *Associated Medical Services, Incorporated: A History* (1987). With the creation of the Institute the AMS endowed it with the funds, capability and responsiblility to develop and disseminate a body of medical history hitherto hidden in the country's memory.

A grants and personnel support program enables the Institute through medical, social and political historians to become a powerful influence in the rapidly expanding interest accorded to medical history. A chair in the history of medicine is supported at each of the five Ontario medical schools.

Originally the Institute's support was limited to Ontario, but it has now been extended to medical historical work in any part of Canada.

Dr. Donald R. Wilson, President of Associated Medical Services, persuaded the Board that the Hannah Institute should launch a series of biographies of those who, as yet unsung, had made major contributions in the broad field of Canadian medicine during their lifetime. The Institute also had in mind for the series members of the nursing profession, particularly those who had pioneered public health services, as well as workers in related fields.

The series opens with the story of Duncan Graham, a determined reformer who became the first Sir John and Lady Eaton Professor at the University of Toronto. Later volumes will record the lives of other Canadian doctors and nurses notable for their scientific, social and political contributions. Biographies in preparation include Joe Doupe, William Mustard, Harold Segall, William Carson, Earle Scarlett, Edward Archibald, R.G. Ferguson, K.G. McKenzie, James M. Langstaff, Marguerite Carr-Harris, Emily Stowe, J.C.B. Grant and William Canniff.

There is no shortage of meritorious subjects. Willing and capable authors are difficult to acquire. The Institute is therefore deeply grateful to the early authors who have already committed their time and skill to the series.

T.P. Morley
Series Editor
1988

CANADIAN MEDICAL LIVES NO. 1

Duncan Graham

Medical Reformer and Educator

by
Robert B. Kerr, M.D.
and Douglas Waugh, M.D.

Series Editor: T.P. Morley, M.D.

Contents

To All Those Who Received Training

in the

Department of Medicine,

University of Toronto

from

Duncan Graham

1919-1947

PREFACE

Modern medicine in North America, with its miracle drugs, organ transplants, synthetic viscera and the like, is a phenomenon of the twentieth century, and most of this has come to us since World War II. The serendipitous empiricism of medical practice in the nineteenth century gave way only slowly to the scientific medicine of today.

In Canadian medical schools at the beginning of the century students were taught to practise medicine through careful observation of their patients, aided only by a few simple and usually crude laboratory tests. The systematic study of disease, rather than just patients, whether in humans or animals, was conducted by a mere handful of ill-equipped scientists working in a few isolated laboratories.

The shift in emphasis from observation and description to scientific study was slow and, like human progress in other fields, was vigorously resisted by adherents to the entrenched conventional wisdom of the majority of both patients and physicians. We do not know precisely when or where this shift began in Canadian medicine but we can identify the major events in its evolution and the individuals who were instrumental in bringing it about. Dr. Duncan Graham was one of them.

The ferment of change in North American medicine did not begin with the pivotal study of medical education in the United States and Canada that was carried out for the Carnegie Foundation by Abraham Flexner and published in 1910. It did however receive its strongest stimulus from that study.

Flexner's indictment of medical schools was succinct, pungent, and devastating. He deplored the slack or non-existent admission standards, the poor quality of teaching, the deficiency or absence of laboratories, the meagre hospital facilities for bedside teaching and, most important, the virtual absence at most schools of research based on scientific methods.

By 1920 many of the worst medical schools had been closed and those that survived were beginning to introduce the changes Flexner had recommended.

Major changes in medical education, as in anything else, are never easy to bring about and can only occur when there is a happy conjunction of circumstances, events and people. Such a conjunction existed at

the University of Toronto at the end of World War I. First, in addition
to the Flexner report, there was a uniquely far-sighted academic
administrator in the person of the university president, Sir Robert
Falconer. Second, there was an exceptionally wise and prescient
chairman of the Board of Directors of the Toronto General Hospital, Sir
Joseph Flavelle. Finally, there was on the medical faculty the extraordinary Dr. William Goldie whose enthusiastic acceptance of Flexner's
recommendations was coupled with an astute perception of the need for
philanthropic support to propel the medical school into the era of
scientific medicine. Goldie's friendship with his patients, Sir John and
Lady Eaton, provided a pathway to that support. Finally, there was the
young Dr. Duncan Archibald (Lamont) Graham, a pathologist who had
been well trained in medical science and who was about to finish
honing his medical and administrative skills in the Canadian Army
overseas.

The appointment of the dour doctor to the University of Toronto's
chair of medicine in 1919 was to spur the department and the medical
school into an era of scientific excellence that continues to this day. The
reserved, self-assured doctor almost overnight converted what had
been a sound, but less-than-spectacular department into a training
ground for medical scientists that was to profoundly influence medical
education throughout English-speaking Canada.

Graham began by ruthlessly ridding the department of those who
were unsuited to the implementation of his policies. He then set in place
a program for the post-graduate training of medical specialists that
became a model for the yet-to-be-born Royal College of Physicians and
Surgeons. He organized patient care and teaching in the medical wards
of the Toronto General Hospital with a logical efficiency that had not
existed hitherto. He began teaching his students by challenging their
capacity for logical deductive reasoning. With a patience that seemed
at times to border on indifference he survived the efforts of a committee
of the Provincial Legislature to block and reverse the changes he had
introduced.

Duncan Graham was very much a man of his time. Despite the
social and economic turbulence of the nineteen twenties and thirties,
life in universities was relatively stable and serene. Professors did not
need to concern themselves with student unrest, virtually unknown at
the time. Department chairmen ruled their small fiefdoms as they saw
fit, without oversight of their actions by the multitudes of committees
that abound today. And chairmen, deans and presidents could rest

comfortably in their appointments until they were displaced by death, retirement or incompetence, whichever came first. This made it possible to plan in the long-range sweep of an academic lifetime, rather than in the brief five-year dollops that are now the norm in our universities. So long as good people were appointed to the senior positions in academe, the system worked well. And when a giant like Duncan Graham came along, one could confidently expect, if not miracles, at least wondrous progress.

This book records the life of this remarkable individual who, by the force of his personality, his integrity, and the cold logic of his thinking, transformed Canadian medical education.

ACKNOWLEDGEMENTS

The initial, and most forceful stimulus for the writing of this book came several years ago in the form of a proposal from the late Dr. Robert C. Dickson. Bob Dickson was an old and valued friend of us both and we were much saddened that he did not live to be presented with a copy of the finished work. We are more indebted than we can possibly say for his proposal and for his encouragement during its preparation.

Duncan Graham left little in the way of letters or other memorabilia. Information about him was obtained from relatives, personal recollections, interviews and archives.

Mrs. Mary Hogarth (Dr. Graham's daughter), Mrs. Lorraine Sutherland (Dr. Graham's stepdaughter), Dr. Alan Bruce-Robertson (Dr. Graham's stepson) and Mrs. Ethel Kelly (Dr. Graham's niece) were all most helpful in providing details of family relations and anecdotes. Miss Mary McInroy, the daughter of Dr. Graham's sister, supplied a family tree that had been prepared by her mother. She also recalled memories of her uncle and showed one of us (RBK) the family homestead and the environment of Graham's childhood.

Miss Stella Clutton, Graham's secretary and administrative right arm during most of his tenure as Professor, was able to recall for us a wealth of information about the department and Dr. Graham.

Dr. Walter F. Prendergast, company medical officer for the T. Eaton Company and a friend of the Graham family, was most helpful with information from the archives of the Eaton Company concerning the deed of gift from Sir John and Lady Eaton which established the Eaton chair of which Duncan Graham was the first occupant. Dr. Prendergast also supplied a great deal of information about the Graham family, and especially about their summer home at Sturgeon Lake.

In interview Miss Kathleen McMurrich supplied information about Mrs. Graham's work in rehabilitation and physiotherapy.

One of us (RBK) was particularly fortunate in being able to interview the late Dr. Walter R. Campbell, Graham's first full-time appointee in the department of medicine. Dr. Campbell recalled the early days of the department as well as his experiences with Graham in England in the later months of World War I.

Much material was made available from the University of Toronto Archives through the kindness of the Archivists Mr. David Rudkin and Mr. Harold Averill. Included in this was the war diary of No. 4 General

Hospital during World War I. Professor Charles Hollenberg kindly made available material from the files of the Department of Medicine. Additional material was supplied by Mrs. Eva Ryten of the Association of Canadian Medical Colleges. In the Provincial Archives of Ontario were records of the controversy described in Chapter VI. Dr. John Hamilton, former dean of the Faculty of Medicine, related discussions he had had with Dr. Graham after his retirement from the chair of medicine.

Oral history tapes prepared by the Hannah Institute for the History of Medicine were a source of comments by physicians who had been Graham's students or colleagues.

Professor John M. Norris, Head of the Department of History of Medicine and Science at the University of British Columbia kindly reviewed and made useful comments on an early version of the manuscript. Others who have read and commented on all or portions of the work include Drs. James H. Graham and Fraser N. Gurd, both former executives with the Royal College of Physicians and Surgeons of Canada; Dr. H. Rocke Robertson, Honorary Archivist for the Royal College; Dr. Robert A. Macbeth, Executive Director of the Hannah Institute for the History of Medicine; Mrs. Lois Kerr and Mrs. Sheila Waugh.

It is a special pleasure to express our thanks to the Eaton Foundation and Associated Medical Services Incorporated and the Hannah Institute for the History of Medicine for the provision of financial support.

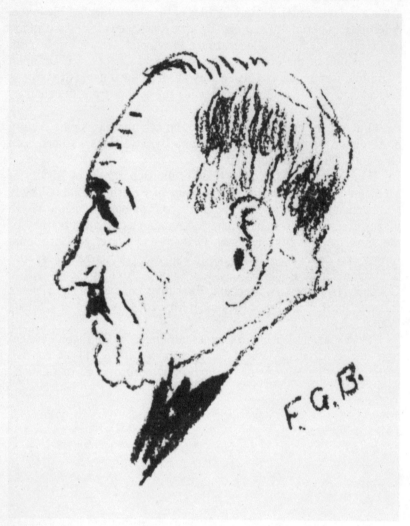

Sketch of Duncan Graham by Sir Frederick Banting.

CHAPTER I
THE CHILD

On January 8th, 1882, Duncan Graham was born in his father's homestead, about a mile from what was then the village of Ivan, in Lobo Township, Middlesex County, Ontario. Middlesex County, in earlier millennia a part of the bed of Lake Erie, now includes some of Ontario's richest farmland. Unlike the sandy tobacco-growing soil of Elgin County on the shores of Lake Erie to the south, the deep black earth of Middlesex County can support all manner of temperate climate crops and livestock.

At the time of Duncan Graham's birth, Lobo was a bustling and prosperous township of 3,500 persons. In both Middlesex and Elgin Counties the farmers were mainly immigrant Scots — McIntosh, McNeil, McArthur, Campbell, Scott, McLean, McKinnon, McKinley, McDougall, McIntyre, McKay and Grahams being the commonest names.[1] Twenty-two of the Lobo Township farmers were Grahams, though not all of them were Duncan's kin or necessarily related to one another.

The first Graham ancestor to settle in Lobo Township was Duncan's great grandfather, Peter, who arrived with his wife, Jane Thompson, in 1828. Already in their early fifties at the time, we do not know whether they had left Knapdale in Argyllshire as evicted crofters, like many Scots migrants of the time, or whether they came, like others, in search of greater liberty and political independence.

Being among the first settlers following the 1820 survey of the township, Peter and Jane, with the help of the three sons and four daughters who had accompanied them from Scotland, had to undertake the exhausting task of clearing the land of its heavy timber before it could be farmed. The family must have found the task rewarding and farm life appealing, since all seven children remained in Lobo Township in their adult years, most as members of farm families.

Peter's son, Duncan P. Graham, married Christina Lamont. She must have been a formidable lady to have had her surname, Lamont, carried forward to two of the sons in her family of ten, and to three of her grandsons. Although her grandson Duncan was christened only as Duncan Archibald, he began as a young man to call himself Duncan Archibald Lamont Graham, possibly to distinguish himself from the multitude of other Duncan Grahams, both in his family and among the many Grahams in the neighborhood. The Scots of that day, as in this, were monotonously unimaginative in the choice of names for their children.

Donald Lamont Graham, Duncan's father, who was known as Dan, had established himself and his wife, Susan on a farm of 1.2 square kilometres which they called "Maplehurst", in the eighth Concession of Lobo Township. The Graham homestead still stands there and, like its neighbours, it is a substantial two-storey buff coloured brick structure, built on a square plan with a slate roof. Its postal address now is R.R. 1, Ilderton, a village in London Township.

The village of Ivan then had a population of about fifty persons and, like others in southwestern Ontario at the time, had a grist mill, a general store, a blacksmith shop, and a church, which was, of course, Presbyterian. The original small frame church which had been built in 1851 was moved in 1861 and replaced by a larger structure in 1886. Its churchyard contains the graves of Duncan's great grandparents, grandparents, and his mother and father, as well as a number of aunts, uncles and cousins. There is also a stone engraved to the absentee "Duncan A.L. Graham, M.D.", whose ashes lie in a Toronto graveyard.[2]

Duncan was the first-born of Dan Graham's four children, being followed by David, Margaret and Peter, twelve years younger than Duncan. The Graham children, like all farm children, were required to do the chores of feeding chickens, milking cows, and bringing firewood to the farm kitchen. Most chores had to be done before breakfast, which was appropriately early. When old enough, they would then set off on the two-and-a-half kilometre walk to Bear Creek school on what is now called Bare Creek Road. The latter spelling doubtless derives from the summer activities in the creek rather than the local fauna.

If the Graham family was like others in the area, virtually all labour on the farm would have been provided by Dan and Susan and their four children. In most years the outlay for hired help would have been nil or very close to it. A judicious combination of livestock and field husbandry spread the demand for labour fairly evenly throughout the year. Field crops were most demanding in the summer when the animals required little attention. In winter, cattle in the barn needed considerable daily labour. Gaps in labour demand were filled with such tasks-of-opportunity as cutting wood, taking grain to the grist mill or spreading manure on the land. The entire cycle was, of course, subject to the merciless unpredictability of the weather, to whose whims successful farmers managed to adopt a "take her as she comes" attitude.

In his book *The Scotch*, also published under the appropriate title *Made to Last*, John Kenneth Galbraith describes in fond detail his recollections of farm life in Elgin County along the southern border of Middlesex in the early years of the twentieth century.[3] Galbraith portrays a hard-working, close knit community of thrifty Scots farmers. Among them were those who regarded children primarily as "valuable earning assets" on whom little should be spent on education and similar frivolities before they were added to the farm's labour force at the youngest possible age. Such families had large broods and both boys and girls were quickly added to the work force. Other families set great store by the merits of education. They tended to have fewer children, whose entry into productive employment was correspondingly delayed. Both Galbraith and Graham had the good fortune to be born into such families although, in each case, earlier generations had been more prolific and less educated. Both Duncan and his brother David went to university. Peter, the youngest, remained on the farm where he became a successful breeder of prizewinning Clydesdale horses.[4]

First-born children are often bright and this was certainly so in Duncan's case. As the eldest child in a farm family he would early have been given responsibilities, including those of tending his younger siblings. Because of this he would have come to occupy a position rather more elevated than the others in management and decision making in family affairs. This, coupled with the aggressiveness that is often seen in those of slight stature such as Duncan's, would have provided an early basis for the skillful tenacity that characterized his later career.

CHAPTER II
THE YOUNG MAN

When Duncan Graham had completed his primary education at Bear Creek school, his parents were sufficiently impressed with his progress to accept the expense of his board in London while he attended the London Collegiate Institute. In four years he finished high school, matriculating in 1901.

As a bright young farm boy we can expect him to have been an interested and possibly speculative observer of the complex biology of crops and animals. While such interests may have led his contemporaries into careers in farming, engineering, agricultural economics or the law, Duncan was drawn to a career in medicine. Whether this was stimulated, as was often the case, by the powerful influence of a family doctor, a mother's ambition, or some other driving force, we do not know. What we do know is that, in electing to go to university, young Duncan was joining an intellectual élite of less than two percent of those who had started school when he did.

He seems to have had no qualms over a decision to enter medicine. Rather than spend a couple of years in an Arts or Science course at university, as many did, he enrolled in 1901 directly from his Collegiate matriculation into the University of Toronto Medical School.

Although the Toronto medical faculty was already one of considerable prestige, competition for admission was not nearly as severe as it has since become. Ten years later young Fred Banting, who went on to discover insulin, was admitted from a general Arts course with quite indifferent grades. Indeed, he had been required to repeat a year because of poor standing, and was allowed to "carry" a failing grade in French which he had to make up later.[1] One cannot help wondering how many potential Nobel laureates are nowadays kept out of medical school by rigid, grade-centred admission standards.

The medical curriculum was similar to that of the better North American schools of the time. There was no requirement for premedical Arts and Science courses. Today's prerequisite courses in chemistry, physics and biology were incorporated as part of the first year medical course. The entire program occupied five years of which the first two were devoted to the basic medical sciences of anatomy, physiology, physiological chemistry, pharmacy and pharmacology, and methods of physical examination. This was followed by three years of pathology, medicine, surgery, obstetrics and gynaecology, therapeutics, jurisprudence and toxicology, contagious diseases as well as instruction in diseases of the eyes, ears, nose and throat, together with hygiene, mental diseases and anaesthetics.[2] Although teaching was mainly in the form of lectures, students in the last three years were required to attend the hospital wards, to witness autopsies, do laboratory and hospital work, and prepare a thesis.

Graham appears to have been an average student who attained distinction neither in failed grades nor in prizes. It was perhaps a portent of his subsequent highly developed flair for administration that he became manager of the varsity lacrosse team and that he organized, as the function's President, the first medical "At Home". This festivity replaced the annual dinner that had been a fixture for many years. Medical student dinners at most universities were then, as now, notoriously rowdy affairs and it is a tribute to Duncan's powers of persuasion that he was able to convince his fellows to adopt the more sedate "At Home", which became an annual event.

A fellow student described him at this time as "Always ambitious...(he) has found time to make many friends...". Another called him "...a man of gifts and graces." The late Dr. Elizabeth Bagshaw of Hamilton, a fellow graduate, says Duncan was "...rather a quiet boy — he never had much to do with girls; he was fond of lacrosse, baseball and rugby. He would sometimes (even) leave college for a day and go off to a game".[3]

When he wasn't skipping classes, playing games or studying, Duncan found time to join his fellow students in activities at the Phi Delta Theta fraternity house. Even if he was a bit shy with girls, he seems, in other respects, to have been a well rounded student who paid attention to both the academic and non-academic activities of the campus.

When Graham received his M.B. in 1905 (it was only in the late 1920s that the University began to call its degree M.D.), scientific medicine as we now know it was quite undeveloped. What little research there was, was mainly in the laboratory sciences, and the most active and exciting of these was bacteriology — a science that had only come into existence a bare thirty years earlier with the pioneer work of Louis Pasteur. Pasteur's discoveries were quickly followed by Robert Koch's identification of the tubercle bacillus and the first "specific" antisyphilis drug, salvarsan, by Paul Ehrlich. These and other momentous discoveries made bacteriology the darling of both the lay and professional press. It is not surprising that the science should have attracted a bright and curious young graduate like Duncan Graham.

Immediately after graduation he applied for and was accepted for the post of Assistant Bacteriologist to the Provincial Board of Health of Ontario. The atmosphere in the laboratory must have been conducive to the exercise of scientific curiosity. During his year in the post, Graham found time from his duties to collaborate with its chief, Dr. G.G. Naismith, in publishing a paper on the haematology of carbon monoxide poisoning and to write independently another on leukocytes and leukocytosis. Both were published the following year. The fact that the papers dealt with haematological topics reflects the much broader scientific base enjoyed by bacteriology at the time.[4]

The following year (1906-7) was spent as resident in the closely related field of pathology at the Toronto General Hospital. During the two years following his graduation Graham also held the position of Don at the men's residence of University College. The Don lives in the university residence and is expected to act as a sort of ombudsman and father-confessor to his charges. He may have chosen to apply for this position in the hope that the experience would help him overcome his reserve in dealing with others.

The next two years were spent in Pittsburgh, where he continued his study of pathology at the Tuberculosis League of Pittsburgh under its Director, Dr. William C. White. During this period he was co-author of three reports on studies of the use of tuberculin in the diagnosis and treatment of tuberculosis.

It was unusual for a North American medical graduate to spend more than a year in training after graduation with the M.D. Of those who did, few spent more than a couple of years in further training. Medical graduates of the day were considered fully qualified to practise medicine, surgery and midwifery, and most proceeded to do just that. There were no certificates of specialization that required mandatory periods of training. The few who, like Graham, went on for higher training were those who combined a healthy scientific curiosity and an equally healthy bank balance, since post-graduate training posts were paid poorly, if at all. Even by modern standards the six year duration of Graham's post-graduate training would be considered lengthy. In the first decade of this century it was exceptional. Many of those who chose this path went on to become the leaders in academic medicine as chairmen of university departments and/or deans.

We don't know whether at this stage Graham had chosen such a career path, although his rate of publication in scientific journals of the day was such as to ensure his coming to the attention of the world of academic medicine. In the ten years following his graduation he published fifteen papers, two in 1907, four in 1909, one in 1910, five in 1911, two in 1912 and one in 1915. His papers dealt with such varied subjects as tuberculosis, haematology, syphilis and poliomyelitis, and appeared in journals published in Canada, the United States, Britain and Germany.[5]

Then, as now, publications played an important role in the advancement of an academic career. Graham's output, in number, quality and diversity would have been bound to attract attention.

It is not known how he supported himself during the two years after he left Pittsburgh when, following in the footsteps of earlier Canadian and U.S. graduates, he went to London, Dresden, Heidelberg and Berlin for further studies in bacteriology, pathology and medicine. It was in Berlin, under Professor Krause, that he gained his only formal post-graduate educational experience in clinical medicine, the discipline in which he was to make his name.

In 1911, at the age of twenty-nine, Duncan Graham returned to the University of Toronto as Lecturer in the Department of Bacteriology, a post he held until 1914, when he enlisted for military service in World War I.

CHAPTER III
SOLDIER-SCIENTIST

The peace of the summer of 1914 was shattered by the assassination at Sarajevo of Austrian Archduke Franz Ferdinand on the 28th of June. Within six weeks Austria-Hungary had declared war on Serbia, Germany was at war with Russia and France, and on August 4th Britain (and Canada), reacting to the German invasion of Belgium, entered the war against Germany.

The distinguished Canadian historian, Arthur A.M. Lower, quotes Lord Morley as saying that he "could imagine nothing less likely than men from some American country such as Canada fighting for the neutrality of Belgium." Yet fight they did, with distinction, and in remarkably large numbers.[1]

Among anglophone Canadians there was no serious debate about the rightness or wrongness of the war. Although it is doubtful that many of them were familiar with, or cared about, the Balkan squabbles in which it had its origins, it was enough that Britain was in it. Ties to the Mother Country were, for many, much stronger and more immediate than they are today.

Duncan Graham responded to the outbreak of war like thousands of other Canadians of his age — he enlisted in 1914. After training with the University of Toronto contingent of the Canadian Officers' Training Corps he was gazetted as a Lieutenant in the Canadian Army Medical Corps in November. He spent the first three months of 1915 as bacteriologist investigating a meningitis outbreak in the military camp at the Toronto Exhibition Grounds.

At about this time No. 4 Canadian General Hospital was mobilized around a core of officers chosen almost entirely from the University of Toronto's medical faculty. In April Graham was promoted to the rank of Captain and joined the hospital as bacteriologist in the laboratory directed by the University's erstwhile Professor of Pathology, Major J.J. Mackenzie. As soon as the hospital reached England in May Captain Graham was seconded as bacteriologist to No. 2 Canadian General Hospital at Le Tréport, a seaside resort on the channel coast of France, where he spent the next four months.

A Canadian nurse at Le Tréport developed a crop of boils which Graham incised. From the pus he made a vaccine from which he gave her a series of injections and the boils subsided. By this time the reserve that had so bothered him a few years earlier seemed to have been at least partly overcome. She recently told one of us (RBK) that "Duncan Graham was quite a gay blade, much sought after by the nursing sisters at dances in the mess."[2]

In mid-October 1915, Graham was returned to No. 4 General Hospital which, four days later, was embarked from Southhampton for the Mediterranean. After stops in Malta and Alexandria the unit was finally disembarked at the eastern Greek seaport of Salonika.

The hospital's role in Salonika was to serve the troops of the British and French expeditionary forces already based there. These forces were by now being reinforced by troops beginning to be withdrawn from the ill-fated campaign in the Dardanelles. The initial intent of the Allied bridgehead in Salonika had been to provide a base from which to reinforce the efforts of Serbia, to the North, in resisting invasion by combined Bulgarian and German forces.[3]

By November the Bulgarian-German armies had succeeded in cutting off the Serbians who managed to withdraw to the west, through Albania and the Adriatic coast, to the island of Corfu. There they re-grouped, re-equipped and, in April 1916, joined the Allied forces in Salonika to await an eventual thrust at the Bulgarians and a return to their homeland.

That thrust was not to come until 1918. In the meantime the allied forces, which now included Italian, Serbian and a few Russian troops in addition to those of France and Britain, remained dug in over a 130 kilometre radius around the port of Salonika. They remained there until September 1918. When they finally broke out they defeated the Bulgarian army, and thus started the collapse that culminated in the final defeat of Germany two months later.

Military historians still debate the wisdom of the allied forces maintaining, and even enlarging, a huge force in Salonika. By the time of the final breakout there were nearly 600,000 Allied troops in the small enclave facing about 700,000 Bulgarians, German troops having by then been almost all withdrawn to the western front. The Germans derisively referred to the Allied forces as "our largest internment camp", or "an enemy army, prisoner of itself." The eventual overthrow of the Bulgarians is seen by many as the ultimate justification for maintaining and strengthening the base in Salonika.[4]

No. 4 General Hospital established a tent hospital of 750 beds on a gently sloping plain, about eight kilometres northwest of the city of Salonika on the road to Monastir. The site provided a fine view of the city of Salonika and on a clear day Mount Olympus could be seen 80 kilometres to the southwest. The arrival of heavy autumn and winter rains turned the site into a muddy morass and in the late spring of 1917 the hospital had to be moved into huts on more suitable terrain.

Immediately on their arrival in Salonika, Major Mackenzie and Capt. Graham set about establishing their tent laboratory, much of which had to be improvised. Water was in short supply and there was no illuminating gas to operate bunsen burners and sterilizers; methyl hydrate or coal oil became less satisfactory substitutes. So successful were they in establishing the laboratory that within a month of setting up it was designated as the central laboratory for all British Forces in the Salonika area.[5] Nothing could have been better calculated to hone Duncan Graham's already well developed medical and organizational skills than the challenging circumstances under which he had to work in Salonika.

With a relatively static battle front and correspondingly few battle casualties, most of the work that he and Mackenzie had to cope with was that generated by an army living in the foul conditions of trench warfare. Their equipment was primitive and often makeshift and their own living conditions but little better than those of the soldiers they served.[6]

Graham's work at this time was mainly in the fields of bacteriology and parasitology. Dysentery and malaria were endemic and the onset of cold weather in early December yielded several cases of frost-bite. This was not unreasonably attributed to the combined effects of freezing weather and the fact that for long periods the men's clothing and blankets were soaked. One soldier's frostbite progressed to gangrene, fatally complicated by tetanus. There were also cases of what was then called "trench nephritis."[7]

In the relatively static battle situation a large proportion of the hospital's patients suffered from the direct or indirect effects of exposure and poor sanitation that is unavoidable in trench warfare. Trenchfoot and pneumonia were particularly common during the winter months, with dysentery and malaria predominating in the summer. Regardless of the season, the flow of bacteriology and parasitology specimens to the laboratory was continuous. Of 2,327 stool specimens that were examined between July and December 1916, dysentery amoebae were identified in seventeen. Bacillary dysentery was much more common than amoebic. Of 1,489 stools that were cultured during the same period there were 403 isolates of what was then called *B dysenteria - Shiga* and 132 *of B. dysenteria - Flexner Y*.[8]

Fighting consisted only of occasional minor skirmishes, so that the volume of medical work was consistently far below the hospital's capacity. It was unusual for more than 500 of its 700 beds to be occupied, and, for much of the time, occupancy was much lower. As a result, hospital personnel had plenty of time on their hands. Certain personnel occupied themselves with sight-seeing in the picturesque antiquities of the city of Salonika. Others, like Major Mackenzie, wrote long letters to their wives, often several each day. As an outlet for professional curiosity and energy the medical officers of the British and Canadian hospitals formed the "Salonika Medical Society" which held regular meetings in one or other of the hospitals. The meetings of the Society enabled its members to maintain and polish their scientific and academic skills in a way that would have been difficult or impossible in a busier theatre of war.[9]

The opportunity was not wasted on Graham and Mackenzie and several others from No. 4 who became regular contributors to the meetings of the Society. One of Graham's presentations consisted of a discussion of the laboratory tests for relapsing fever of which he had seen a number of cases. On another occasion he read a lengthy and detailed paper entitled "Some Points in the Diagnosis and Treatment of Dysentery occurring the the British Salonika Force". In it he effectively linked the clinical and laboratory aspects of this scourge of the fighting troops. The paper was seen by Lt. Col J.G. Adami, Assistant Director of Medical Services for Canadian Contingents and, in peacetime, Chairman of McGill's Department of Pathology. He called it "both the fullest and, in many respects, the most important article written by an officer in the C.A.M.C." In 1918 it was published in the prestigious journal *Lancet*. The journal editorialized, "We commend Major Graham's paper as a valuable contribution to the study of dysentery, and emphasize the practical nature of the hints he gives as to diagnosis and treatment."[10] What is remarkable is that Graham was able to report his study in one of the world's outstanding journals on the basis of work done in an ill-equipped field laboratory that had, for a time, been housed in a tent.

An important advance in treatment of the dehydration of dysentery was the use of saline or glucose solutions injected either intravenously or subcutaneously. Occasionally, however, a patient so treated, instead of improving, went into a state of shock and collapse. Graham was able to demonstrate in experiments with young rabbits that there were no toxic effects of saline infusion; and a colleague, Captain Imrie, noted that reactions could be avoided if saline solutions were made up from chemically pure salt and distilled water rather than with the salt tablets widely used at the time.

Graham's background in bacteriology, his use of the laboratory, not just as an aid to diagnosis but as an adjunct to the study of disease, and his willingness to engage in the limited animal studies that could be undertaken in a military hospital, marked him as one of the small but growing new breed of academic physicians — the group that came to be called physician-scientists.[11]

Major J.J. Mackenzie returned to England in the summer of 1916 and Graham succeeded him as Officer-In-Charge of the laboratory.

Among the enlisted personnel of No. 4 in Salonika was Canada's future Prime Minister, Lester B. Pearson. Pearson and Graham had first met in the Collegiate in London, Ontario, when Pearson was a cadet and Graham a sergeant in the Cadet Corps. At No. 4 Pearson was for a time Graham's batman. Many years later, when the Prime Minister had occasion to visit Graham in his office in the Banting Institute, he stood in the doorway at rigid attention and saluted his former officer.[12]

One of the less scholarly diversions at the hospital was an improvised two-hole golf course. Other entertainment was found in informal parties. At one of these, held in Mackenzie's tent, "Salonika Punch" was served. It was a concoction of hot cocoa laced with whiskey, which Mackenzie described as "a very delicious mixture if you don't put too much whiskey in it...just enough to flavour it. It makes a fine mixture to go to bed on."

Although the Salonika front was relatively static, the Allied shipping in the harbour was periodically bombed by enemy aircraft, which included an occasional Zeppelin. In one such raid a bomb landed on the hospital burying Mackenzie in the laboratory under a cascade of bottles, bedpans and the like, from which he was rescued, unharmed, by Graham.[13]

Graham was promoted to Major in 1917. A few months later No. 4 relinquished its site at Salonika to a British hospital and was embarked for England where it was re-established as a General Hospital at Basingstoke in Hampshire, about seventy-five kilometres southwest of London. In October, Graham was mentioned in despatches for his work at No. 4 Canadian General Hospital.[14]

By this time word of Graham's work in Salonika had filtered back to the University of Toronto where pressure was exerted to have him returned. In October 1917, No. 4's commanding officer, Col. W.B. Hendry wrote to Dr. C.K. Clarke, the superintendent of the Toronto General Hospital and Dean of the medical faculty, quoting Adami's comments on Graham and saying "You will see by this what Duncan has been doing for us. I hear a whisper of a desire to recall him for work at the University. Now this must absolutely not be. He is making a reputation for the University over here and also one for himself. He is now doing some valuable work on 'Trench Fever' and it would be disastrous to have him recalled now or later."[15]

A short time after this, in December, Hendry again wrote to Clarke saying, "Duncan Graham is at present over in France completing his investigation of trench fever which he started in Salonika. I let him go for a period of six weeks and expect him back about the middle of January."

Amid a rising tide of rumours, Graham was shifted from No. 4's laboratory and named as Officer-in-Charge of the hospital's Medical Division in June 1918 and promoted to Lieutenant-Colonel. By this time the hospital had expanded to two thousand beds and with it, Graham's responsibilities. But the pressure to have him return to his *alma mater* continued to mount.

CHAPTER IV
DR. GOLDIE: KINGMAKER

At the time of Duncan Graham's return to the University of Toronto in 1919, medical education in North America was in a state of rapid, often turbulent change. In Toronto this was reflected by developments that created unique opportunities for an aspiring academic physician of Graham's bent and background.

Since the turn of the century medical education in the U.S. and Canada had been emerging from its earlier pattern of trade-school apprenticeship into a more formal academic model of sound university standard. The shift was most striking at schools like Johns Hopkins, Harvard, Columbia, Pennsylvania and Michigan in the United States, and was beginning to be felt at McGill and Toronto in Canada.[1]

Although the transition to medical programs of university calibre had begun to be evident by 1900, it received its most powerful boost from the definitive report of Abraham Flexner — *Medical Education in the United States and Canada* — published in 1910. The report was based on Flexner's visits to each of the 155 medical schools that then existed in Canada and the United States. He found much to criticize and little to praise, and his comments were nothing if not both cogent and pungent. The report's honest, often brutal frankness gave it almost instant credibility.[2]

The Flexner Report has been described variously as "a journalistic tour de force," and "a classic of muck raking journalism." Within a decade it had become widely accepted as the prescription for medical education in the two countries.[3]

Flexner favoured the development of clinical departments under full-time professors within a proper university setting. He promoted close integration of the basic and clinical sciences and the application of the scientific method to practice as well as to research. He scorned didactic teaching and favoured instead learning by doing. Another of Flexner's tenets that was particularly germane to the Toronto situation was his insistence that the medical school control its teaching hospitals. Although Flexner found the schools at Toronto and McGill to be first class, both, at the time, fell short of his stringent criteria of excellence as, indeed, did most of the schools in North America. The introduction of the Flexnerian model of medical education at the University of

Toronto came about largely due to the efforts of five extraordinary individuals: Joseph Flavelle (later Sir Joseph), Sir Robert Falconer, Dr. William Goldie, and Sir John and Lady Eaton. These five were the principal architects of the emergence of the medical faculty into its golden years of post-Flexnerian excellence.

Joseph Flavelle, whose pork-packing company was the largest in the British Empire, was, by 1902, sufficiently secure in business to be able to devote more and more of his time to public service. In that year he joined the Board of Trustees of the Toronto General Hospital and two years later became its chairman. With the support of Mr. P.C. Larkin, another newly appointed board member, Flavelle instituted a wide-ranging reorganization of the hospital's housekeeping and laboratory services.[4]

Clinical teaching at the time had been conducted at both the General and St. Michael's Hospitals on a quite informal basis. Flavelle decided that the General Hospital should become an exclusive, or "closed" teaching hospital. Both he and Larkin recognized the unsuitability of the Gerrard Street site of the hospital for its long-term development in such a capacity, and they shortly set about searching for a more suitable location.

In spite of vigorous opposition from Toronto City Council and from many practising physicians, Flavelle was able to engineer an agreement in 1906 between the Hospital and the University whereby the University would acquire a 3 hectare parcel of land on the south side of College Street, an area on which a new hospital building could be erected. The hospital in turn agreed to convey to the University a block of land on the north side of College Street to accommodate the departments of Pathology, Bacteriology and Pathological Chemistry, and other departments, as might be required. The lands were duly acquired and the new 670 bed hospital, at the time the largest in Canada, was opened in June 1913. The marriage between the interests of the hospital and those of the university satisfied one of Flexner's most important requirements.[5]

The provincial government's Toronto General Hospital Act of 1911 provided that hospital medical staff appointments would be made on the recommendation of a Joint Hospital Relations Committee. The by-law respecting medical staff provided that "all public ward patients shall be entered under the care of heads of services and shall be available for clinical instruction of students of the Medical Faculty of the University of Toronto."[6]

This formal fusion of the interests of the Hospital and University was greatly facilitated by the presence on the Hospital's Board of

Robert Falconer (later Sir Robert), who had become president of the university in 1907. Falconer was a Presbyterian clergyman and classics scholar who had been educated at London and Edinburgh Universities. He has been described as an unemotional and cerebral scholar. During his presidency he brought about the merging of a collection of colleges into an integrated university.[7]

By 1919, when Dr. Alexander McPhedran, the University's Professor of Medicine and Senior Physician at the General Hospital, retired, at the age of seventy, from both positions, Sir Robert had an intimate acquaintance with the complex inter-relationships of the two institutions. He took personal charge of the search for McPhedran's successor, relying heavily on the advice of Dr. William Goldie.

Goldie, a medical graduate of Toronto, was one of those shadowy figures who exert a powerful influence on the events of their times without themselves seeking, or being thrust into, positions of prominence and power. A bachelor, he had served under McPhedran as chief of the hospital's medical out-patient service. By the century's second decade he was at the peak of his career, a much respected clinician and one of the wise men whose counsel in the affairs of the Faculty and Hospital was often sought and usually heeded.

Goldie was a strong advocate of the system of full-time clinical appointments that had been proposed by Flexner. He appears to have had little difficulty in persuading Falconer that McPhedran's successor should be a full-time appointee rather than being required to subsist, as McPhedran had, on his clinical earnings, with an insignificant honorarium from the University.

It was one thing to persuade the University President what was needed, but quite another to find the means of its accomplishment. This Goldie was able to do through his friendship with the Eaton family, to whom he was personal physician. The head of the family, Sir John Eaton, had, in 1907, assumed direction of the T. Eaton Company, the country's largest and most profitable department store chain. Sir John was already a major benefactor of the Toronto General Hospital and was favourably disposed toward both the Hospital and the medical faculty.

He had met Flora McCrea, the future Lady Eaton, while he was a patient at the small private hospital where she worked as a student nurse. This happy medical experience seems to have provided a lasting basis for the interest that both the Eatons were to show throughout their lives in the Hospital and the Medical Faculty. It is not therefore surprising that they should have responded favourably to Goldie's proposal.[8]

In his discussions with Sir John and Lady Eaton, Dr. Goldie told them that, if the University and Hospital were to have an outstanding department of medicine, it was essential that an endowment be provided to support a full-time professor who could devote his entire effort to the development and administration of the department, free from the demands of a busy practice. The Eatons agreed to donate $500,000, to be made available in annual payments of $25,000 over a period of twenty years. The magnitude of the Eaton's generosity can only be fully understood by recognizing that the purchasing power of the dollar in 1920 was at least twenty times what it is in the late 1980s.

The letter of acknowledgment that Sir Robert Falconer sent Sir John in May 1918, although replete with Scottish restraint, makes canny reference to his perception of the needs and expectations of the new chair:

> Mr. Walter Wiley and Goldie both spoke to me about your splendid intention with regard to the development of the Department of Scientific Medicine in the University of Toronto. If you decide to carry your present intention into effect I am sure that you will develop a department of the University which requires large funds in order that it may be placed on a basis equal to that of the leading universities of the United States, which will make it possible to train medical men who will enjoy advantages in Toronto second to none anywhere. Of course the equipment of the Faculty of Medicine means that the whole body of the people throughout the length and breadth of this land will be beneficiaries.
>
> I think you will agree with me, and I have no doubt that the committee would that a gentleman of the status whom you hope to have appointed would have to be given a free hand for a period of years with regard to the organization of the department, and that in the main it would have to be left to him to decide the details of the expenditure of his department, provided always before he has been appointed the general outlines for the expenditure of money have been agreed upon; that is to say, how much in general should be devoted to Scientific Medicine proper, and how much to Paediatrics.[9]

The reference to "large funds" was doubtless intended to ensure that Sir John realized the importance of long term planning and financing. The reference to the "free hand" to be given to the "gentleman of the status whom you hope to have appointed" was, as we shall see, to give rise to repercussions that were probably more violent than either Sir Robert or Sir John could have foreseen.

Sir Robert's letter went on to say that the University's Board of Governors would authorize him to name a committee to cooperate with Sir John in choosing a nominee for the appointment. He proposed the names of Dr. Goldie, Dr. Alan Brown (Physician-in-Chief at the Hospital for Sick Children), Dr. B.P.Watson (Chairman of the Department of Gynaecology and Obstetrics), Dean C.K.Clarke and himself. It is clear from the tone of the letter that Sir John was to have a major role in making the appointment.

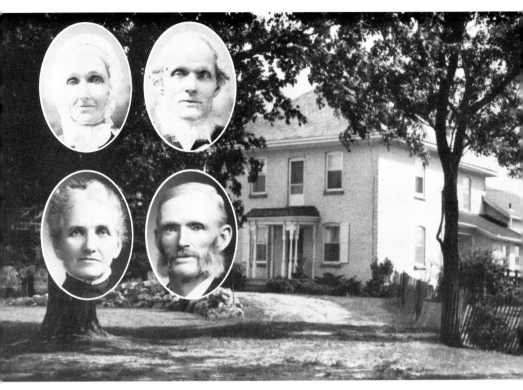

*Graham homestead at Lobo Township, Middlesex County, Ontario.
Inset, clockwise from upper left, are Christina Lamont Graham,
Duncan Graham's (DG's) paternal grandmother; Duncan P.
Graham, DG's paternal grandfather; Donald Lamont ("Dan")
Graham, DG's father; and Susan McDonald Graham, DG's mother.*

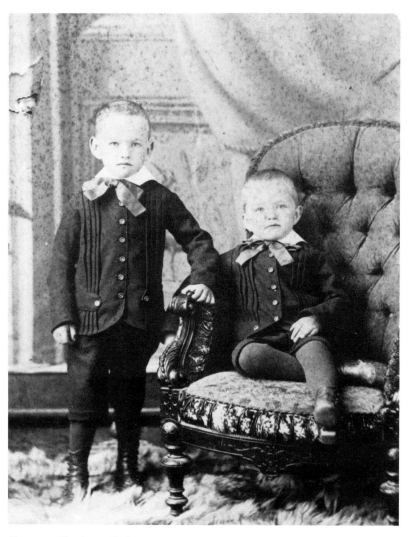

Duncan Graham (left) and brother David, circa 1886.

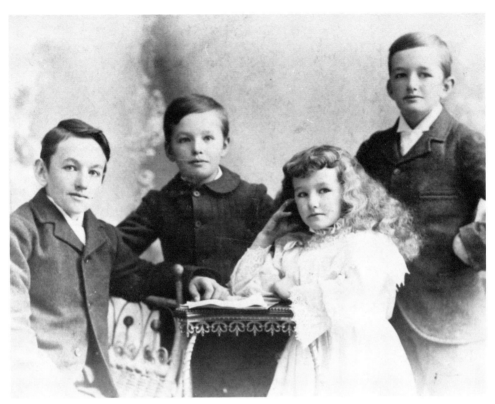

From left to right, Duncan Graham, Peter, Ethel (sister), David (brother), circa 1890.

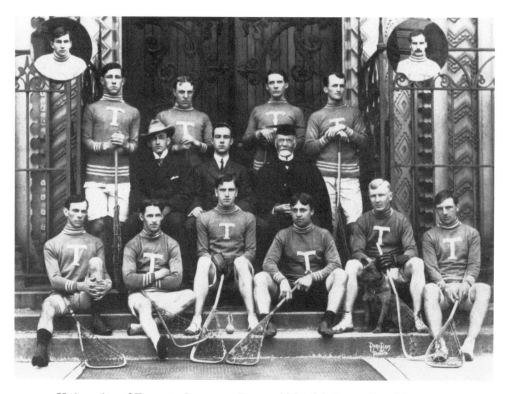

University of Toronto Lacrosse Team, 1905-06. Team President
Duncan Graham, in fedora hat, led his team to the North American
Intercollegiate Championship of that year.

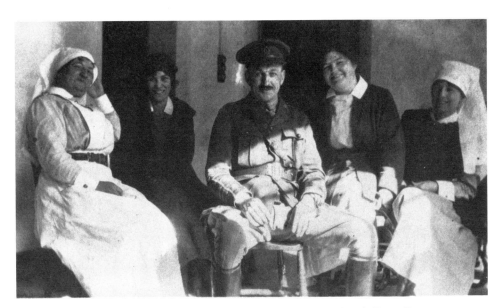

Captain Duncan Graham with Nursing Sisters, No. 4 Canadian General Hospital, Salonika, 1915-17.

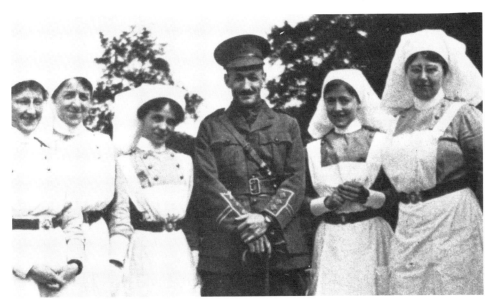

Graham with Nursing Sisters, No. 4 Canadian General Hospital, Salonika, 1915-17.

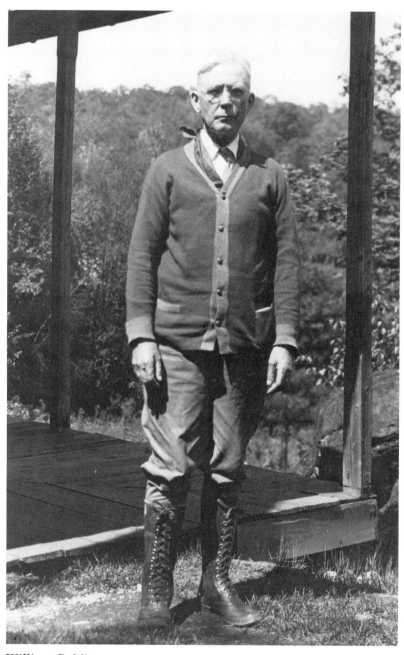

William Goldie

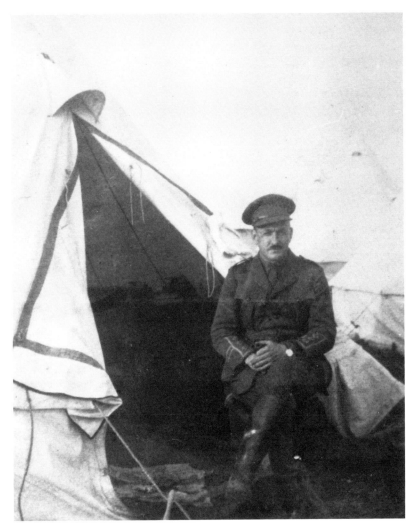

Graham in Salonika, 1915-17.

Ethel Graham McInroy,
Duncan's sister.

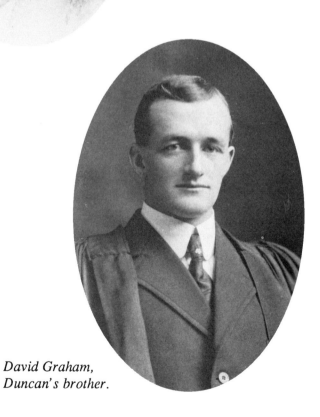

David Graham,
Duncan's brother.

CHAPTER V
THE SEARCH

The search for a candidate to fill the newly created full-time chair began in May 1918. One of the first candidates put forward was Goldie himself, whom Dr. Alan Brown had nominated to the Eatons. Goldie promptly declined it. He himself proposed a Dr. Hewlett of Stanford University, a candidacy that does not appear to have been pursued.

Dr. Goldie had recently enlisted in the Canadian Army Medical Corps and was about to join No.4 General Hospital at Basingstoke. President Falconer directed him to join with Duncan Graham and Professor Leathes, the Dean of Medicine at the University of Sheffield, in seeking possible candidates in England and Scotland. Leathes, who, before returning to Sheffield, had occupied the chair of Pathological Chemistry at Toronto for five years, was a familiar friend of the Toronto Faculty.

Goldie sailed for Britain in July 1918, where he joined No. 4 General Hospital at Basingstoke. In September he wrote to Sir John, "I had a chance to size up the pathologist Duncan Graham, with a view to proposing his name to the President if he should fail in his attempt to secure T.R. Elliott or H.H. Dale."[1]

President Falconer, who was also in England at this time pursuing the search, was unable to persuade Elliott to consider leaving England's war-depleted medical professoriate. Elliott chose instead to accept the professorship at University College Hospital in London. Falconer was similarly unsuccessful in interesting Professor H.H. Dale (later Sir Henry) who was already Director of the Wellcome Physiological Research Laboratory and who went on to a distinguished career as Director of the National Institute for Medical Research. It is clear from the calibre of candidates being considered that Falconer knew that, thanks to the Eaton benefaction and the favourable academic climate in Toronto, he was in a position to seek out the very best candidates.

Goldie was pessimistic about the possibilities of recruitment from the United States. "The outlook for first class men from the U.S. is very poor, though a search will be kept up until the spring, at least."[2]

He arranged for Falconer to visit Basingstoke to meet with himself, Leathes and Graham to discuss the principles that should govern the

Department of Medicine. The four found themselves in remarkably close agreement. Their discussions undoubtedly focused on the "full-time" concept and the desirability of laboratory and basic science applications in clinical medicine. They would also have talked about the promotion of clinical research and undergraduate and post-graduate teaching. Graham clearly made a favourable impression during these meetings. Leathes said of him, "I am ashamed that I had not thought of him as a possible candidate, he is the type that is required — an organizer, an administrator and wonderfully fitted by his clinical and laboratory training to stimulate research and the training of young men on the staff."[3]

Falconer, however, had some doubts, mainly that Graham was too young. He tried to persuade Goldie to reconsider his earlier refusal, "taking the appointment as a cover for Graham for a few years." Goldie pointed out "the absurdity of this plan" and once more refused.

At about this time Goldie became a strong advocate of Graham's candidacy. He wrote to Sir John: "In the unit here he is not only respected but liked even though he is an exacting task-master. He can say 'No' — and does not lack for tact. He has one fault and he does not allow it to blind him to the good points in another — he never forgets meanness or a lack of frankness. The more I see of him the more do I believe that he could carry the plan to success."[4]

Goldie's letter appears to have had the desired effect for on November 16, 1918, five days after the signing of the Armistice, Sir Robert wrote to Goldie telling him it had been agreed to offer the position to Duncan Graham. He went on to say that Sir John and Lady Eaton "had made inquiries of their own and were convinced that he was the man."

Falconer asked Goldie to talk to Graham "to find his views and try to persuade him to accept. You may say that we shall endeavour also to secure in the hospital such an arrangement that he will have full control of all materials he needs for teaching purposes. Very probably we shall be able to secure a change in the matter of medical services and have them under the direction of one man, at least we will attempt to secure this."[5] His uncertainty was indeed portentous.

Graham's response to these overtures, relayed via Goldie, was that he would accept the position only if Goldie had excluded himself and if he were given a free hand with respect to the staff; "...such would be equivalent," wrote Goldie, "to the resignation of all members of the Department."[6]

It is curious that these negotiations should have been conducted in this roundabout way, with Dr. Goldie as intermediary serving both sides. Such a procedure might have been appropriate if there had been tricky and sensitive points to be ironed out, but this seems not to have been the case. Perhaps Falconer simply wanted to keep Goldie in the picture to ensure that he was on side to support Graham when the need arose. Such a feeling seems have been mutual, since Graham suggested that Goldie should return to Toronto as soon as possible, with Graham to follow soon after. Whatever the case, Goldie in fact returned to Canada in January.

On January 10 Sir Robert wrote to Graham stating:

> ...our Committee ... unanimously decided that you should be approached.... You have been so strongly supported not only by Goldie but by Leathes, Watson and several others that our Committee has unanimously come to the decision. I may say that Sir John and Lady Eaton, after having made independent inquiries were in favour of you. ...Details as to salary, expenditures and relations to Paediatrics have not yet been worked out by the Committee, but we are asking to have Dr. Goldie brought here in order to work the details out before the final appointment is offered to you. ...You must be gratified to know that those who have associated with you and who are acquainted best with your work are most strongly in support of your appointment.[7]

Graham responded:

> I beg to acknowledge the receipt of your letter of Jan. 20th informing me that my name had been the unanimous choice of the Committee appointed to consider possible occupants of the new chair in medicine.
> The knowledge that my associates in medical work were the strongest supporters of my name, although affording me the greatest cause for personal gratification gives me an increased consciousness of the responsibility of the position that I am being offered.
> After your letter to Dr. Goldie I discussed with him the conditions under which I could accept the appointment. His knowledge of the conditions will aid you and your Committee in the discussion of the details which you mention in your letter as being necessary for consideration before the final appointment is offered me.

If I receive the appointment I should like to begin my work about the middle of May, i.e. before the present session ends.[8]

Clearly both Graham and Sir Robert had implicit faith in Goldie as their intermediary.

Dr. Walter R. Campbell says that in the spring of 1919 the curiosity of the officers of No. 4 General Hospital was aroused by the fact that "all the Professors of Medicine in Britain and lots of eminent people" visited the hospital. Particular note was taken of visits by Dr. Goldie and President Falconer. Eventually Graham told Campbell that "It will appear in orders tomorrow that I am leaving to become Professor of Medicine in Toronto." After accepting Campbell's congratulations Graham urged Campbell to return with him to Toronto. As it turned out Campbell had to remain in Basingstoke where, while awaiting his repatriation orders, he arranged the purchase of apparatus for his Toronto laboratory in anticipation of the staff appointment Graham had promised him.

Duncan Graham's appointment was announced by President Falconer on April 28, 1919, to take effect on July 1. At about this time Sir William Osler, who was then Regius Professor of Medicine at Oxford, wrote to Falconer: "Graham's appointment has been very well received over here, and I am asking all the Professors of Medicine in the United Kingdom to meet him next week at dinner at the Athenaeum." This was a particularly generous gesture, since Osler heartily disapproved of the kind of full-time appointment to which Graham was going.[9] In a letter to the President of Johns Hopkins University in 1911 he had referred to "this cruel Whole-time Professor experiment."

I cannot imagine anything more subversive to the highest ideal of a clinical school than to hand over young men, who are to be our best practitioners, to a group of teachers who are *ex officio* out of touch with the conditions under which these young men will live.... As students of the wide problems of social reform so closely associated with disease, the clinical men should come into contact with the public, whose foibles they should know, and whose advisors they should be.[10]

Osler was indeed the quintessential clinician who reflected the best traditions of astute bedside observation and correlation of clinical and laboratory findings. But his attitude to full-time teachers was out of date. The new breed of Flexnerian clinician had a more scientific view of medicine and used the laboratory not just to assist in clinical diagnosis but to study disease itself.[11] Shortly before his death in 1919, Osler's attitude seemed to have changed. He wrote to McGill's Dean of Medicine to propose that the new Professor of Medicine at that school should have control of appointments in the teaching hospitals and that the full-time system be introduced in the Departments of Medicine, Surgery and Gynaecology at the two hospitals — the Montreal General and the Royal Victoria.[12]

CHAPTER VI
CLEAN SWEEP BY THE
NEW BROOM

From the developments recounted it might seem that young Duncan Graham's ascent to the chair of medicine at the University of Toronto in May 1919 had been so well planned and prepared that a smooth transition of the Department into the new era of scientific medicine was inevitable.

The favourable academic climate included the fact that at Toronto, as at virtually every other medical school in North America, the Department of Medicine was the largest and strongest component of the Faculty. It had the most powerful impact on medical education as well as on patient care. The Eaton gift assured the Department of stable financial support at a handsome level for the foreseeable future. Sir John and Lady Eaton had prudently seen to it that support from the University would not be diminished because of the gift. At $13,000 per year this support was substantial.

Of the Department's total annual revenue of $38,000, $10,000 was to be allocated as salary for Dr. Graham and a further $5,000 was earmarked as support for the Division of Paediatrics, which, though based at the Hospital for Sick Children, was to continue to be a responsibility of the Department of Medicine.

The close integration of the interests of the University and the Toronto General Hospital that had resulted from the negotiations between Flavelle and Falconer had created the kind of climate favoured by Flexner. The University already had the strong, scientifically-based departments in the basic medical sciences: anatomy, physiology and biochemistry, pathology, and pathological chemistry, all of which Flexner had considered essential. The fact, however, that all hospital staff appointments were the responsibility of the Joint Hospital Relations Committee and that all public ward patients were to be available for teaching was not, in fact, as ideal an arrangement as it might have been.

The "heads of services" referred to in the hospital bylaw were the heads of the three "coordinate services" in the Department of Medicine. (There were four in Surgery.) These services were actually autonomous so far as treatment of patients was concerned and were also, to a very large extent, independent of one another in their teaching activities.[1] Each service was a fiefdom of its director. There was no preselection of patients by disease category. Furthermore, as elsewhere in Canada and most of the United States, there were no agreed standards for the qualification of specialists and no established training programs for specialists and potential faculty members.

Until 1919 members of the clinical teaching faculty served the University voluntarily or were rewarded by small stipends that were little more than tokens. Under the circumstances it is surprising that the quality of the teaching was considered to be very good. Although an appointment to the clinical faculty of the University brought little or no direct financial reward, it was nonetheless highly valued by its possessors. Academic rank brought prestige, which in turn brought patients — and that meant income. Thus any change that threatened the security of academic ranks or positions of authority such as headships of coordinate divisions could be expected to generate vigorous and prolonged resistance.

It may have been in anticipation of such problems that the terms of the Eaton gift stipulated the creation of a committee to advise the President of the University on the reorganization of the Department of Medicine and, in particular, on expenditures of departmental income. Then, as now, it was advisable to have decisions that were likely to prove unpopular made by a committee, rather than by an individual.

In any case, Duncan Graham wasted no time in imposing on the Department the changes he had negotiated with the University and the Hospital. By mid-July he had persuaded the advisory committee to approve the replacement of the "coordinated services" at the Toronto General and the Hospital for Sick Children with a single service in medicine and to dispense with all designations of rank within the Department save for those of the Head of the Department, and for Drs. William Goldie and Alan Brown, who were to be Associate Professors. All others were to have the same rank as "Clinicians in Medicine." All ranks were to be renewable annually, as indeed they had been in the recent past.[2]

The singling out for special status of Goldie and Brown, who had been members of the search committee, does not appear to have bothered either Graham or Falconer. Brown's appointment placed him in charge of Paediatrics, which may have been sufficient justification in his case. Goldie, however, had played a pivotal role in Graham's appointment and it is surprising that his appointment did not provoke outraged cries of "patronage." That they did not is doubtless a reflection of the high regard in which Goldie was held, both as a clinician and as a wise advisor.

Graham also proposed that the small honoraria paid to clinical teachers be discontinued and the money be used instead for departmental maintenance and to provide full-time salaries for those he intended to appoint in that capacity. He wrote to the President, "I have discussed this question with the men I have interviewed re: appointments in the Department and have explained the reasons for advising this. I do not look forward to any particular trouble should this be acted upon by you."[3]

In unifying the department under the Professor, who was also the Hospital's Physician-in-Chief, Graham created three ward services in the public wards. Instead of random admission to these services, as had been the case with the coordinate divisions, each service was made responsible for specific categories of disease. The Ward G service was for neurological, haematological and dermatological diseases, Ward H for metabolic, endocrine, rheumatic and gastrointestinal disease, and Ward I segregated patients with diseases of the heart and lungs.

By late September 1919 the Board of Trustees had approved Graham's nominations to the Hospital's medical staff. Conspicuously absent from the list were seven of the eight former Associate Professors, including Major-General J.T. Fotheringham who, as Director General of Army Medical Services, had approved and facilitated Graham's early return to Canada. The others were Associate Professors A. M. Baines (Paediatrics), W. B. Thistle, R. J. Dwyer, H.B. Anderson, J. Graham Chambers, J. Ferguson; Associate in Clinical Medicine W.J. McCollum; Demonstrators in Clinical Medicine E.C. Burton, B. O'Reilly, C.J. Wagner, C.S. McVicar, G. W. Ross, R. W. Mann; Assistant in Clinical Medicine T. G. Glover. With the stroke of a pen Graham had revoked the appointments of nearly forty percent of the Department's staff.[4]

CHAPTER VII
A STORM OF PROTEST

The radical organizational changes that Duncan Graham introduced were sufficient in themselves to generate a storm of protest from those who were affected. They were shortly joined by unhappy surgeons who had been similarly dealt with by the new head of that Department, Dr. Clarence L. Starr.

Starr, who had just succeeded to the Chair of Surgery had been, like Graham, appointed full-time Professor, in this case with the financial support of the Rockefeller Foundation. He followed Graham's lead in replacing the four coordinate services with a single service under himself as Surgeon-in-Chief.

It can have surprised no one that such radical changes in the organization and staffing of the two major clinical departments of the city's largest hosptial led to a row. Criticism began to appear in both the professional and public press, directed at the President and Board of Governors of the University, the Trustees of the Hospital and, of course, the two Professors themselves.

Particularly vigorous criticism was directed at the "involuntary retirement" of General Fotheringham, Dr. (Lt. Col.) Chambers, and Dr. (Maj.) Thistle in the Department of Medicine and Dr. (Col.) J.A. Roberts, Dr. (Capt.) A. Moorhead , Dr. (Capt.) J. McCollum and Dr. (Col.) Herbert A. Bruce of the Department of Surgery. The critics took particular glee in pointing out that all these men were below the "statutory age limit", whereas two of those whose appointments had been renewed in the Department of Surgery, Drs. Alexander Primrose and G.A. Bingham, were past the limit.[1]

Physicians of the day were as ponderously long-winded as they are now when aggravated. An editorial in the *Canadian Journal of Medicine and Surgery* stated:

> So it was in the early stages of this controversy that the President was sharply criticized for not exercising his authority in preventing the dismissal of certain gentlemen from the staff, who, it was declared, should not have been dismissed, and the retention of others who had passed the statutory age limit. An expression commonly heard was

that his actions were 'autocratic in the extreme'; and it was further added, that he neither permitted the voluntary retirement of these gentlemen slated for dismissal, nor did he acknowledge the debt of their service to the university over many years in an academic capacity, or pay tribute to them as military surgeons in the Great War. The axe was raised, and he permitted it to fall (so went the allegations!).[2]

An editorial in the *Canadian Practitioner Review* was directed at Duncan Graham:

> The appointment of a young and inexperienced laboratory man, be he ever so competent in research, to be whole-time Professor of Medicine in the University of Toronto, with unlimited powers in the choice of the staff of medicine, has occasioned deep grumblings and rumblings. These have resounded through the halls and wards of the Toronto General Hospital, an institution closely associated with the clinical and laboratory work of the medical student. Some excellent and experienced men have resigned never to take up clinical teaching again. Toronto is not supremely blessed with proficient teachers in medicine at the present time. Death, sickness and overseas and military service have caused a thinning of the ranks. Many men profess to see disaster to a great institution which a few years ago counted its able clinicians almost by the score. The Government must look alive or they will have both hospital and university tumbling about their heads. That medicine has not yet arrived at the time when the experimenter takes supersedence over the clinical diagnostician and the therapeutist, many aver, the laboratory man to the contrary notwithstanding.[3]

Further fuel was added to the fire of protest by a letter that President Falconer circulated to members of the clinical staff. In it he pointed out that a condition of the gifts from the Eatons and from the Rockefeller Foundation was that the Governors should spend no less money in the departments concerned than they had hitherto. Since, by March 1920, the Faculty had committed itself to developments that would require funds beyond those generated by the combined revenues from the gifts and departmental budgets, his letter went on to say that the Board of Governors had approved the discontinuance of the teaching honoraria, so that the money could be used for salaries. These salaries were to be provided to "such staff in the Clinical Departments as are not dependent for their living on private practice and are giving all or nearly all their time to the work of the university."[4]

By January 1922, when objections from the staff had begun to diminish, the controversy was rekindled by Col. Thomas Gibson, a decorated war veteran and University of Toronto alumnus who was Assistant Deputy Minister for Militia Overseas. Gibson made public a demand for an investigation of the whole affair. The government responded by appointing a Special Committee of the Provincial Legislature to "inquire into the organization and administration of the University of Toronto, including its relation with the Federated Colleges and with the Toronto General Hospital." The Committee was given power to subpoena and to take evidence under oath, and was under the chairmanship of the Premier himself, Mr. E.C. Drury.[5]

During the next sixteen months the Committee held fourteen hearings. So seriously did Sir Robert Falconer view the proceedings that he was in "continuous attendance." Presumably he kept both Duncan Graham and Clarence Starr up to date on the proceedings since neither of them either asked or was invited to meet with the Committee.

Certain of the physicians who appeared before it used the occasion to castigate the University for endangering the status of the "family doctor" by training too many specialists, and to criticize the system of education as being "ultrascientific" rather than practical. Critics with similarly anti-intellectual sentiments can still be found, sixty-five years later. They may be less numerous but they are no less vocal.

Others, like Dr. George W. Ross, a discontinued Demonstrator in Clinical Medicine who had served on one of the "coordinate services" under Dr. Graham Chambers, whose appointment had also been terminated, directed his criticism at the organizational changes. In his testimony to the Committee he said "there has existed and one wonders whether there does not still exist what might fairly be termed an obscure influence, an elusive something, that has exhibited a certain liveliness from time to time." He continued:

> By what influence were those in authority induced to permit the abolition of the three coordinate services in medicine and the four in surgery in the Toronto General Hospital and the substitution of one head for each, contrary

to the Act? ...Finally, is there any explanation for the virtual dismissal of certain distinguished members of the medical and surgical staff of the Toronto General Hospital, during the reorganization, who were under age and the retention of others who had passed the statutory age limit?

"These dismissals were illegal," he said. "...As far as I am aware the Act has not changed and yet these services were abolished and one head was appointed for Medicine and one for Surgery."[6]

With a twist of the rhetorical knife he noted that three of the dismissed men, General Fotheringham, Col. Chambers and Col. Rudolph were serving their country in the Army when the reorganization was announced.

It may have been on the advice of his lawyer that he finished his diatribe stating:

If I have had the occasion to refer to individuals or bodies of men in authority and perhaps to criticize their acts, I should like to disclaim any thought of imputing wrong or doubtful motives to anyone, for it is not difficult to understand that high minded men, upon occasion, may commit acts ostensibly for the good of the state or of an institution to which they are devoted, which would not have been condoned in any private or personal relationship and knowing as I do the gentlemen concerned in the matter I have discussed, I have no hesitation in accepting the explanation which, at the same time, I may not be prepared to acknowledge it as sufficient justification.

Dr. H.B. Anderson, whose appointment had not been renewed and who had had a role in the original establishment of the three coordinated services, complained to the Committee, "We have one man at the head of the department, and he is in control of the patients not only at the General Hospital, but ... St. Michael's, the Sick Children's and the Western Hospital ... the new system limits initiative and the opportunity for independent work....it is an organization...on business rather than academic lines...that is contrary to a democratic idea of hospital or university government."[7]

One of the more eloquent and influential critics of the new organization was the suave and persuasive surgeon Dr. Herbert A. Bruce, who was later to become the province's Lieutenant Governor.

Bruce, whose appointment in surgery Dr. Starr had terminated, wisely confined his criticism to principles rather than personalities. He warned the Committee against too much of a swing to the laboratory and mechanical side of medical practice and the neglect of observation and personal diagnosis. He opposed the principle of full-time professorships and deplored the expenditure of public funds on such an experiment.

Not all the critics of the new order whose appointments had been terminated were malcontents. Dr. K.C. McIlwraith, an Associate Professor of Obstetrics, criticized the way in which the Council of the Faculty was constituted. In a twist of reasoning that may have made some sense at the time, he said that there were too many men of Scottish descent on the Faculty, adding, ominously, "this might prove unhealthy to university development."[8]

Another obstetrician, Dr. F. W. Marlow, also objected to the full-time professorship. His scattergun criticism was that it commercialized the teaching of medicine, increased spoon-feeding of students, led to excessive standardization, eliminated fair competition among teachers, increased costs, and centralized authority.

Not all of those appearing before the Committee were critical of the new organization. Sir Joseph Flavelle, responding to those who objected to the increased emphasis on science, pointed out that nine-tenths of the men who were teaching were in fact practising physicians or surgeons "at the bedside of patients every day." To this, committee member and, as it turned out, next provincial Premier, the Hon. George Ferguson responded, "You shatter this whole case." Dr. W.E. Gallie, at the time on the surgical staff at the Hospital for Sick Children and who later became Professor of Surgery and Dean of the Faculty, told the Committee he strongly favoured the full-time professorship concept.

One of Graham's stoutest defenders was his predecessor, Dr. Alexander McPhedran, who told the Committee that, if the new program were carried out, Toronto's medical faculty would be an example to the world. He pointed out, not entirely accurately, that many places in the United States were following the Toronto example — Harvard, Yale, Columbia, Washington, St. Louis, San Francisco, Chicago, Iowa City, Indianapolis, and he said that McGill had also adopted the plan. He told the Committee that in the autumn of 1922, at the Royal Canadian Institute, Dr. George Vincent, President of the Rockefeller Institute, had said "nowhere was the background for scientific and practical medical training as good as in the Toronto General Hospital." It was McPhedran's opinion that, under the former system of three separate services, such advance would have been quite impossible.

Amid the tumult of claim and counterclaim over the merits and defects of Graham's reorganization, the instigator of the fuss kept to himself. There is no written record that he played any role in the debate, nor that he attempted to influence any of the protagonists. He seems to have chosen to let his actions speak for themselves, apparently confident that the inherent wisdom of his decisions would be vindication enough.

Whatever Duncan Graham's expectations were of the legislative committee's inquiry, he can have found no cause for joy in the report it presented to the Legislature in May 1923. The report took the side of the University's critics in almost every case. It had nothing good to say about the reorganization of the Departments of Medicine and Surgery, which it castigated as "illegal and unauthorized." It went on to say that "no Order-In-Council should now be passed confirming what was irregularly done...". The report deplored the fact that the staff at the Toronto General Hospital was "controlled absolutely by the university, and no member of the medical profession not on the university staff may attend patients in the hospital except in the private and semi-private wards ... a condition (which) is undesirable." The present University-Hospital agreement should be abrogated, the report said, and a new agreement entered into and validated by the Legislature.

The Report had similarly unkind words for the terms of the Eaton and Rockefeller endowment provisions which facilitated the appointments of single heads in medicine and surgery, and for the liquidation of the positions of the coordinate heads. "The Committee has no hesitation in saying that in a publicly-owned University, private endowments shall not be accepted if, attached to them, are conditions which would bind the University Governors to any particular policy or course of action."

These concerns and recommendations were embodied in a Draft Bill for an *Act to Amend the University Act* which was appended to the report. Under the Bill, the University Senate would be required to "approve the terms of proffered endowments before acceptance of such endowments by the Board of Governors."[9]

We can only speculate on the impact that the committee report might have had if any part of it had been adopted and acted upon by the Government. It is clear that the Committee rejected many of the progressive principles that were embodied in the Flexner Report and that were promoted under the terms of the Eaton and Rockefeller grants. The Committee's report in fact constituted an endorsement of the *status quo* and a repudiation of President Falconer, the University's Board of Governors and the Hospital's Board of Trustees.

We could find no record of the reactions of these bodies to the report, nor of the sentiments it may have engendered in Duncan Graham, Clarence Starr or other central participants in the planned reorganization. This is not entirely surprising since the unfolding of events left little time for any reaction. Ten weeks after the report was tabled in the Legislature, the government of Premier Drury was defeated, to be succeeded by a Conservative regime under the Hon. George Howard Ferguson. Ferguson, as we have seen, had been a member of Government's Special Committee where he had been favourably impressed with Sir Joseph Flavelle's spirited defence of the University's new regime. It doubtless came as no surprise to the protagonists in the controversy that Ferguson's government chose to leave the report mouldering in the files, bureaucrats eventually sending it to the Provincial Archives where it rests to this day, undisturbed by itchy legislative fingers.

Duncan Graham's role as a silent spectator of the entire debacle would thus appear to have been justified. He cannot, however, have been entirely complacent at so close a brush with a destiny that could have overturned his plans and catapulted the medical school backwards into the preceding century.

CHAPTER VIII
THE PROFESSOR'S NEW PROGRAM

The controversy generated by Duncan Graham's appointment did not inhibit him from proceeding immediately to introduce changes in the department staff, its educational program and its sense of direction.

Though diffident and gentle by nature, Graham had by now learned to have confidence in his own skills at organization. He was untroubled by the self-doubts and vacillation to which many educators are prone. He was, as we have seen, supremely confident in his own judgment and had the toughness to put his ideas into effect. His opinions were honest and forthright, to the point that they occasionally led to misunderstandings that generated antagonism. On the whole, however, the logic of his straightforward reasoning, which was deductive rather than intuitive, persuaded almost all with whom he worked of his unshakable integrity and honesty. He was a man who generated enormous respect, admiration and even devotion, if not always warm affection.

The new professor proceeded immediately with the appointment of additional full-time faculty. The first of these was Dr. Walter R. Campbell, who had had extensive experience in biochemistry under Professor A.B. Macallum. His special competence was with the analytical methods related to metabolic and endocrine disorders, for which he was given responsibility in the Hospital's public wards. Next came Dr. H.K. Detweiler who was made responsible for the development of serologic procedures, especially the Wasserman test, and for allergic disorders. Dr. Ross Jamieson was appointed in cardiology and Dr. Norman Keith in what is now called nephrology. Keith soon left the department to join the staff of the Mayo Clinic.[1]

It was Graham's plan that those chosen for membership in his department would spend two or more years as full-time appointees giving major time and effort to research and teaching as well as to public ward patient care. Later they could revert to part-time or volunteer status and develop private consulting practices. Convinced of the importance of the laboratory basis for clinical medicine, Graham organized a course in clinical microscopy for undergraduate medical students, under the supervision of Dr. G.W. (Stony) Lougheed. The course emphasized instruction in laboratory methods, with special focus on haematological diseases.

Even though Graham's own training and experience had been almost entirely in the laboratory he saw to it that, not only in his own teaching, but in that of others in the department, strong emphasis was laid on history-taking. And, to ensure that students became aware of the social context of disease, he arranged for final year students, under supervision, to see patients in the out-patient department. Even in the 1980s medical student experience in ambulatory care is considered deficient at many North American medical schools. Graham's emphasis on it in the 1920s, while not unique at the time, reflects a keen and prescient appreciation of its importance.

Dr. Graham's philosophy of medical education was carried forward into the still unorganized field of post-graduate education of trainees in internal medicine. Although there were at the time no national standards for the training of medical specialists, Graham set forth his views in a letter to President Falconer: "Postgraduate laboratory training in one of the departments of Physiology, Pathology, Bacteriology, and Serology or Pathological Chemistry is considered essential in the preliminary training of all graduates entering the department of Medicine as prospective teachers of clinical medicine in the future."[2]

It was one of Graham's most strongly-held views that clinical medicine in academic centers could only prosper and advance if junior members of the staff were protected, through substantial salary support, from the demands of practice for a sufficiently long period to develop their skills in teaching and research. This remained his policy throughout his 28 years as Head of his department. In this dedication to a system of full-time appointments, with limitation on professional practice, he joined the new wave of medical education in North America. It was a clear break with the Oslerian tradition of teaching based on practice rather than on the research laboratory. Graduates (and their successors) of similar programs are the modern clinical scientists who conduct research and train graduate students in their own laboratories. This has reduced or eliminated the demand for the training in departments of the basic medical sciences that were so important in Graham's day.

Duncan Graham never developed a large clinical practice. Although he maintained a private office separate from the University and Hospital to see referral patients, he never permitted this practice to encroach on his time for academic effort.

It is likely that a major reason that the report of the Drury Commission was never acted on by succeeding governments was the almost immediate success of Graham's new program. Under his unified system of departmental management the assessment of student progress became more rational and uniform. The segregation of hospital patients by disease category made both teaching and patient care more efficient and effective, and was quickly appreciated by both students and staff. Dr. George S. Young , in his testimony before the Drury Commission, extolled these advantages and emphasized that this was "certainly not in the direction of ultra-scientific medicine....The student graduating in medicine ... was never as well qualified to meet the problems of general practice in country or town as he is today."[3]

One of Graham's innovations was not successful and had to be reversed. He had underestimated the resistance that would be generated by his decision to cut off the honoraria of clinical teachers. A committee appointed by President Falconer to review the Department of Medicine's programs recommended that the honoraria be reinstated, and this was acted on by the Board of Governors. The Committee also softened the impact of the dismissals of staff members in Medicine and Surgery by urging the Dean and the heads of departments to show every possible consideration to individuals who had given service to the university and who might have been adversely affected by the reorganization of the departments.[4] There is no record, however, of the form this "consideration" took. It seems likely that the entry in the minutes was intended to soothe the conscience of the Committee rather than to heal the wounded pride of the dismissed faculty.

As a teacher, Duncan Graham's impact on both undergraduate students and the resident staff was profound. His small wiry frame, his slim, stern, usually unsmiling visage gave an impression of rigid inflexibility that was softened only by the twinkle in his eyes of amusement or approbation. In private, students and staff rarely referred to him as "Dr. Graham." To them he was "The Professor," "The Prof," "Dunc" or "The Old Man". One class nicknamed him "The Brow" because the natural furrows in his forehead became accentuated as he raised his eyebrows when questioning a student.

Graham's approach to teaching and, indeed, to all aspects of life can be appreciated by recognizing his devotion to what he called "the discipline of science." To him science was based in logic and he sought always to find a pure and continuous thread of logic in any situation. Once he had satisfied himself that the thread was continuous and unbroken he neither needed nor sought any further basis for conviction.

His convictions, thus formed, were unshakable and untroubled by doubts.

His teaching was normally carried out in a lecture room in the form of theatre clinics for third and fourth year students, and at weekly ward rounds on each of the three medical services. His principle method was that of Socratic dialogue, in which he peppered students with questions, often starting with "Why...?". Students accustomed to the more didactic lecture form of teaching were disconcerted by Graham's emphasis on logically based deductive reasoning. Since he often focused persistently on one or two students who fell within his line of sight, his classes quickly learned evasive manoeuvres. These consisted in placing themselves so that the central rows of seats that fell directly under his gaze were vacant — a positioning the football buffs referred to as "The Graham Formation." Dr. Irwin Hilliard, a former student and trainee, says Graham was mercilessly harsh with students who made silly statements or who failed to provide logical support for their clinical conclusions. Not all students were able to recognize that such criticism was simply an exercise of Graham's own logical processes and had no basis in personal vindictiveness.[5] Graham was delighted when a student or resident could turn the tables on him in logical argument.

In 1936 a young woman with streptococcal meningitis had been treated with Prontosil, the first sulfonamide, of which Graham had acquired a few precious vials. The interne who presented the patient to Dr. Graham was Dr. Peggy Blenkin, daughter of the Bishop of St. Alban's in England. She simply said that this was a case of meningitis cured by Prontosil.

"How do you know it was the Prontosil?" Graham asked her. "You don't suppose that God might have had anything to do with it?"

"Well, Sir, I thought of that," she replied, "but of ninety-seven cases of streptococcal meningitis admitted to this hospital in the last twenty years, God had a chance but He failed in every one." Graham was delighted with this riposte.

Graham's great strength and singleness of purpose could not have brought him success without the enthusiastic support of his department staff and of the central university administration. This he clearly had in abundance. Within the Department he continued to rely on the wise counsel of Dr. William Goldie and Dr. John Oille, with whom he regularly played bridge at the York Club . He also consulted regularly with the four full-time staff members and, most significantly, with Sir Robert Falconer, whose support was reliably firm and continuous.

CHAPTER IX
BANTING AND INSULIN

The opposition to Duncan Graham's appointment had not yet subsided when an even more momentous event thrust itself into the Professor's world. During the winter of 1921-22 a young surgeon, Frederick G. Banting, working under the direction of Dr. J.J.R. Macleod, the University's Professor of Physiology, discovered insulin. Banting had been assisted by Charles H. Best, one of Macleod's graduate students. The two of them found that extracts of pancreas contained something that lowered blood sugar levels in dogs made diabetic by surgical removal of the pancreas. They accomplished this after a series of frustrating, mainly unsuccessful, animal experiments. By January 1922, with the help of biochemist, Dr. J.B. Collip, they isolated a pancreatic extract that could be tested in diabetic dogs and humans.[1]

Few, if any, medical discoveries of this century have had a greater impact on medical care than the discovery that was made in the dingy laboratory that Macleod had been able to provide. Banting, who was a surgeon, untrained in science, had resisted and often resented the guidance of Macleod, the professional scientist. He also distrusted Collip, whom he suspected was trying surreptitiously to patent the discovery.

Like the protagonists in Ben Traven's "Treasure of Sierra Madre,"[2] the four members of the research team were torn by jealousies and suspicions that at times came close to blows. While Banting and Best remained friends, relations between Banting and the Macleod-Collip duo deteriorated permanently and irrevocably.

Graham was drawn into the controversy as the Physician-in-Chief at the Toronto General Hospital, where he had delegated responsibility for the care of diabetic patients to Drs. W.R. Campbell and A.A. Fletcher. He decided that Banting, a surgeon who had never treated diabetics and who was not currently in practice, was not qualified to conduct research on human subjects. Although Graham's judgment was sound, it earned him only suspicion and resentment from Banting. This reaction was aggravated by the knowledge that Graham was friendly with Macleod, whom Banting perceived as a spurious claimant for honours in the discovery of insulin.

Banting's perception of a Macleod threat to steal credit for the discovery of insulin was real and he spoke of it to many of his colleagues. When Graham learned of this he had conversations with both Macleod and Banting and, with help from Banting's friend and surgical mentor, Dr. Clarence Starr, was able to get the two men together and to extract an apology from Banting. Although Banting and Macleod never became friends, Graham's sensitive and diplomatic intervention at this critical point made it possible for the two to continue to work together.[3]

After the encounter of January, Macleod persuaded Graham to allow the first clinical test of insulin to take place under Campbell and Fletcher on the diabetic ward of the Toronto General Hospital. The patient was a desperately ill fourteen-year-old charity patient named Leonard Thompson. On January 11, 1922 Banting and Best had to wait outside while the first injection of an extract prepared by Banting and Best was administered by Campbell's house physician, Dr. Ed Jeffrey. This initial injection resulted in only marginal improvement in Thompson's condition.

Twelve days later an extract prepared by Dr. J.B. Collip proved much more effective. The boy's blood and urine glucose levels fell sharply. Acetone disappeared from the urine. These biochemical gains were accompanied by noticeable improvements in the patient's clinical state.

It was on this threshold of triumph that the clash between Banting and Macleod was aggravated by a news story in the *Toronto Daily Star* in which Macleod was quoted in a way that struck Banting as an assertion of claim on the discovery.[4] At the time, and for many years, Banting viewed Graham with distrust on account of his friendship with Macleod. His sensitivity to what he perceived as the machinations of others bordered on the paranoid.[5]

In January 1923, when Banting, Campbell and Fletcher reported their experience in treating 50 diabetic patients in the *British Medical Journal*, they concluded their article saying, "To Dr. Duncan Graham, Professor of Medicine, we desire to express our sincere thanks for his interest in directing and supervising the investigation throughout its course."[6] The journal, editorializing on the work said, "Statements of this kind are naturally received with caution and even with some misgiving. The reader is bound to ask whether the authors have possibly been misled by their own enthusiasm." It then goes on to say, "But the facts remain that these six patients are alive, that the improvement which was apparent clinically was confirmed by the laboratory data, and that the observations have been made under the supervision of so skilled and careful a clinical worker as Dr. Duncan Graham, Professor of Medicine at Toronto."[7] Although it was a common practice at the time for a professor's name to be appended to papers coming from his department, whether or not he had participated directly in the research, Duncan Graham refrained from attaching his name to any of those early papers on insulin that set the medical world on its ear.

Sixty-five years later we believe the credit for the discovery of insulin should indeed have been shared amongst the principal players in the drama. Clearly the primary credit belongs to Banting, without whose idea and stubborn persistence, even when misguided, the work would not have been successful. Banting, however, could not have prevailed without the laboratory facilities and guidance of rigid scientific discipline provided by Macleod. The work would otherwise have been unlikely to gain acceptance in the world of science. Best, though the most junior member of the team, was essential to its success, not only in providing technical expertise, but, more important, in helping Banting to stabilize and control his volatile temper and to lift him from depression when things were not going well. Finally, the efforts of these three would have come to nothing had not Collip's biochemical wisdom enabled him to purify a potent, clinically effective, pancreatic extract.

The story of the discovery of insulin has been well told by Michael Bliss in *The Discovery of Insulin* and *Banting: a Biography*.[8] Each of the heroes of insulin was engagingly human. Banting was volatile and scientifically untutored. Macleod was such a rigid disciplinarian he was unable to establish the necessary human contact with Banting. Collip, like Macleod, was a scientific disciplinarian, probably the best scientist on the insulin team,[9] who was also unable to achieve a comfortable working relationship with the volatile Banting. Best, the most junior member, joined literally on the toss of a coin and proved himself, both then and later, the most effective team player.

Duncan Graham's role in the insulin story was the vital one of orchestrating the initial clinical testing and eventual introduction to routine patient care. We can imagine the doubts and misgivings that must have beset this dedicated and painstaking clinical scientist on first encountering Banting. It is difficult to conceive of two individuals less alike: Banting, rumpled, robust and impetuously informal; Graham, dapper, slight and fastidious. Graham's initial reaction was to reject Banting's application to treat diabetic patients on the medical wards at the Toronto General. He doubtless saw in Banting the kind of physician of which he had rid his department as soon as he took it over — a man whose training was insufficient and of the wrong kind, who had no experience and little knowledge of the management of diabetic patients. In the cold logic of Graham's mental processes there could have been but one answer.[10] On the other hand, there was the compelling argument of Macleod that the pancreatic extract was indeed so promising as to merit clinical testing. Graham then agreed that insulin could be tested at the Toronto General, but only under the control and supervision of Drs. Campbell and Fletcher. This is where the matter rested, at least for a time.

In February 1922, Banting and Best published "The Internal Secretion of the Pancreas" in the *Journal of Laboratory and Clinical Medicine* in which they described their animal experiments.[11] The following month Banting, Best, Collip, Campbell and Fletcher published the first report on the use of insulin in human patients.[12] In April, the federal government put Banting in charge of a special diabetic clinic at the Christie Street Military Hospital. Since at that time he had access to greater supplies of insulin than Campbell at the Toronto General, Christie Street became the principal centre for the clinical use of insulin.

In *The Story of Insulin* Banting says, "Things were stalemated. Best and I had control of the production of insulin and I had the clinic at Christie Street Hospital and had more private patients than I knew what to do with. So I decided that the Department of Medicine and the Toronto General Hospital could not have insulin for use on its wards until I had an appointment on the staff."[13] Although Bliss questions whether Banting and Best could have adopted and enforced "such a ruthless, ethically questionable position," insulin *was* indeed made available for use at the General Hospital.[14] Meanwhile, Graham, concerned over the welfare of the Hospital's patients, continued to oppose Banting's appointment.

By this time, only a few weeks after the initial publication on the use of insulin in humans, Banting was beginning to receive attractive offers from centres in the United States. The prospect that both he and insulin might leave Canada forever suddenly loomed.

The situation clearly called for prompt and decisive action by the University and the Toronto General Hospital. The only logical agent for such action was Duncan Graham. Accordingly, in June 1922, he asked the Hospital's trustees to consider the establishment of a diabetic clinic. He proposed setting aside sixteen beds on the second floor of the

Private Patients' Pavilion, with laboratory space and equipment, the provision of nursing and orderly staff, and the appointment of a dietitian. In addition, he proposed that public patients with diabetes be cared for on Ward H.[15]

Graham was named Director of the Clinic, with Drs. Banting, Campbell and Fletcher as members of the attending staff. In this way an uneasy truce was established between Banting and the Department of Medicine. Graham continued to have reservations about Banting's clinical knowledge of diabetes and insisted that Campbell and Fletcher have primary responsibility for most of the management of patients. Writing about the situation in 1940, Banting says: "It did not work out well. Graham was a close personal friend of Macleod's. I could tolerate Fletcher but I could not tolerate Campbell. Graham was always absolutely fair and unselfish and I respected him because of his unselfishness and absolute honesty. But we were not friends. I could not talk to him. We did not understand each other. I hated him and he hated me. He was my new chief and though I hated him I played the game with him. I gave him every letter from every single diabetic. I accepted not a single diabetic for private treatment and although it was difficult, I withheld publication of results of treatment of the patients at Christie Street until after the publication of the first report of the patients in the clinic."[16]

Thus Duncan Graham's scrupulous honesty and fairness were responsible for reducing a tempest to a mere state of turbulence, and Banting remained at Toronto. Banting's early grudging respect for the head of his department mellowed over the years, so that by 1940 he was able to write:

> This all seems curious now after these years. I hate to write it but it must be told if the whole truth is to come out. Through the years this same Professor Graham has become the most trusted and intimate of friends. There is no one from whom I now seek advice so urgently and so frequently. Nor is there one on whom I place so much reliance. It is to be noted that I always found him absolutely honest and unselfish and though we had battles because of difference of opinion and now I say we may still differ in opinion but that respect for honesty and unselfishness which I have always had for him will keep us friends. There is nothing that he will do that will ever cause me to distrust the inner man ....[17]

In a further statement that provides insight into both his own and Graham's character he wrote: "In still later years when I was in dire trouble his pronounced and announced faith in me was of the greatest help. In trouble one finds who are one's true friends. He was too Scotch to say a single word to me but he acted what he felt and he said it to others. I only wish that I had known Professor Graham in the early days of insulin as I know him now."[18]

The reversal in the relationship of the two men is the more remarkable when it is recognized that Duncan Graham was then, as he remained throughout his life, a reserved, dour, supremely self-confident disciplinarian, not given to close friendships. Something of Banting's child-like enthusiasm for the loves and hates of life must have penetrated Graham's reserve. The change was real and the affection between the two men was deep. When the bomber carrying Sir Frederick, as he had become, crashed in Newfoundland in 1941 it was Graham who broke the news to Banting's wife.[19]

CHAPTER X
THE DEPARTMENT GROWS AND EVOLVES

It was common practice among medical school department heads of the day to run a department in an autocratic, authoritarian manner. Duncan Graham was no exception to the general rule. He was unencumbered by committees and, although he would from time to time seek advice and opinions from others, it was clear to all that he was the one who made the decisions and took responsibility for them.

When Graham offered the chief resident post to one of his third year trainees, the candidate asked if he should submit an application.

"Hell! No," said Graham. "They haven't turned down one of my recommendations yet, and I'll be damned if they will now."

Whatever the faults of the system of autocratic management, and there were many, in the hands of a skilled operator like Graham it made for speedy, efficient and highly responsive administration. It is doubtful that a modern-day department chairman, encumbered by departmental, faculty and university committees and by the demands for "accountability" at all levels, could have so quickly brought about the radical changes that Graham accomplished within the first months and years of his appointment.

As we have seen in Chapter VIII, Graham quickly reorganized undergraduate medical teaching by segregating patients according to diagnosis, thus ensuring that students were taught by teachers with particular interests and knowledge. He also introduced training in laboratory methods, which to him was the bedrock of clinical teaching and practice. Whether by example, persuasion or edict, others on staff quickly adopted Graham's teaching technique of " Socratic dialogue." Though not unique to the department in Toronto, its emphasis under Graham profoundly influenced other schools, many adopting it in one form or another.

It would be misleading to suggest that Graham single-handedly carried his department and the faculty into its era of post-Flexnerian excellence. In fact, a comparable wave of change was under way at the same time in other clinical departments, most notably in the Department of Surgery under Dr. Clarence Starr. The drive toward scientific medicine and the evolution of the clinical scientist, which had begun to permeate the faculty as a whole, must have strengthened the hands of its directors among whom Graham was but one of the leaders.

Although the changes in undergraduate medical education introduced by Graham were not particularly radical, they demanded changes in attitude among the department's staff. Graham seems to have brought this about, at least in part, by firing many of those who would have opposed the changes. Others were either persuaded by Graham's powerful logic, or perhaps intimidated into changing their ways and outlook by contemplating the fate of their former colleagues.

If the changes in undergraduate education represented nothing more than the application of sound pedagogic principles, Graham's policies in postgraduate training were indeed a radical departure from former practices. As we have noted earlier (Chapter II), there were at the time no national or other generally accepted requirements or standards for the postgraduate education of medical specialists. Graham set about to change this, first within his own department, but later, as we shall see, in the establishment of national standards for the entire country.

Almost immediately after taking over the Department, he established a policy which required a period of four or five years' training after graduation from medical school. Such training had to include at least one year in a basic science. The best trainees who completed this program were then eligible for appointment to the available positions on the Department's full time staff. They would remain in these fully salaried positions for three to five years. During this period of extended apprenticeship, the junior staff member was expected to be heavily engaged in teaching and research, and to supervise patients on the teaching wards. A very limited amount of private practice was also permitted.

At the end of this period, junior staff members' salaries were reduced to the level of a stipend and they were permitted to expand their private practices, while continuing to teach and work on the wards. It was expected, most often correctly, that such individuals, when reverting to "part-time" status, would continue to be active in research and other scholarly work.[1]

It was not until after his retirement, in his 1954 address to the Dalhousie Medical Faculty's Annual Refresher Course, that Graham stated the policy that had guided him in the development of his department.[2] He said then that the Head of a clinical department should be

... constantly on the lookout for potential teachers among his students ... In his seeking for potential teachers for further education and training in clinical science, the Head should select students with character, integrity, intelligence and a liberal education; students who in their daily work display a curiosity to know and understand, and, above all, have a love of mankind. None can exhibit these qualities of heart and mind in full measure, but the clinical teachers must possess them in an appreciable degree, for students learn much by example and precept from their teachers. Medicine is an art as well as a science, and its graduates are members of a learned profession which has been given a code of ethics by Hippocrates, the Father of Medicine, a code to shape their conduct as helpers of mankind.[2]

Even though stated in this florid manner, it is clear that this was the path in which Graham believed and which he followed throughout his career.

While it might have been expected that such a rigorous and demanding program was unattractive to graduates anxious to establish themselves in practice as soon as possible, such was not the case. The demand for enrolment in the Graham program rose rapidly and those of its graduates who were not subsequently appointed to the department staff were quickly snapped up by other medical schools, both in Canada and in the United States.

Within two years of taking over the department, Graham had established both undergraduate and postgraduate training programs that were to persist with only minor alterations throughout his twenty-eight years in the chair.

From the people who knew and worked with Graham during his years as Head of the Department of Medicine we gain a picture of an austere martinet. These comments are from his contemporaries and trainees: "Certainly no one could forget Duncan Graham. He was very tough ... a wonderful organizer. There was no doubt in anyone's mind who was boss."[3] "Graham projected no warmth ... he didn't mean to instil fear but (he) did."[4]

Not everyone agreed about Graham's talents as a teacher. He was "a terrible lecturer. Lectures were an exercise in clinical logic — Socratic dialogue ... he didn't spare the criticism."[5] "Graham taught well if you listened. He was a good example of being kindly to patients, always asked the patient's permission before examining them on rounds ... would warm his stethescope in his hands. (He was a) hard man to get to know — austere, critical (he) embarrassed a lot of people ... was misunderstood."[6] Dr. Irwin Hilliard says that Graham "knew his residents well and followed their progress with interest and a certain amount of affection — which we didn't find out until much later. (We were) all frightened as undergraduates, lectures were question and answer, (we) ended up with few notes and some of the students who looked for notes felt his lectures were a waste. (He was) very critical of nonsense. Sometimes you felt it was a little harsh on the person who made the silly statement but there was nothing personal in it. He felt that medicine was a very logical process of coming to sensible conclusions. Something that was silly (had to be) pointed out very clearly. In this way he didn't endear himself to students."[7]

As early as 1923 Dean Primrose, a respected senior surgeon and colleague of Graham from Salonika days, said in his Annual Report:

> The best evidence of the success of the reorganization of the clinical departments is found in the remarkable activity and enthusiasm displayed within these departments. The clinical teaching is co-ordinated and systematized and has reached a high standard of efficiency such as has not hitherto been attained. The students respond in a manner highly satisfactory, their work is more thorough and comprehensive, they evince an interest and concentration of effort in their work which is admirable. One of the striking features of our present organization is noted in connection with the activities of the staff. They have shown remarkable interest in their staff meeting which has proved one of the most valuable innovations under the present system. The most noteworthy feature of the results attained, however, is the extraordinarily large number of problems of research which have been successfully undertaken by members of the staff and which have added valuable contributions to the practice of scientific medicine. The present organization of the clinical departments has further resulted in marked increase in efficiency in the standard of service rendered to the hospital patients.[8]

A year later Professor Henry Christian of Harvard Medical School, who had been Visiting Professor in Graham's department, wrote, "I have come home stimulated by what I saw in Toronto. You and your colleagues should feel proud of your department. I am sure you are giving your students remarkably fine training. I liked very much the way you are doing the trick there."[9] That this was not just the effusiveness of a bread-and-butter letter was made clear when, following the discovery by Minot, Murphy and Castle at Harvard of the effectiveness of liver treatment for pernicious anemia, Harvard invited the University of Toronto and three other American schools to join in a cooperative study of the effectiveness of liver extract. Mrs. John A. Stewart of Perth, Ontario, donated the magnificent sum of $15,000 to the Department to support this project.

Graham can only have been elated when in 1923 the Nobel Prize in medicine was awarded to Banting and Macleod. The university promptly honoured its Nobel laureates with honorary degrees, but refused Banting's request to confer the same honour on Best. That omission was at least partly corrected in 1930 when the University opened the Banting Institute, across College Street from the Toronto General Hospital, in which generous accommodation was provided for the Banting and Best Department of Medical Research. The Institute also housed the Departments of Pathology, Pathological Chemistry, student laboratories and lecture theatres, as well as providing offices and laboratories for the departments of Medicine, Surgery, and Obstetrics and Gynaecology. Medicine occupied much of the building's third floor. It was not until 1950 that the University opened the Best Institute next door to the Banting to house the Department of Medical Research.

Stella Clutton, Graham's incomparable departmental secretary for twenty-five years, recalls that when the Department moved into the Banting Institute, Graham told her that, now that they were near the hospital, she was to maintain an open door to students and residents. It was Stella herself who became that open door, skillfully calming apprehensive visitors who, as often as not, were terrified at the thought of an encounter with the formidable "Prof."

In 1932 the University's Board of Governors decided to name the Chair of Medicine "The Sir John and Lady Eaton Chair of Medicine."[10] In 1936 paediatrics was finally made independent of Medicine as a separate Department. It continued, however, to receive the annual grant of $5,000 from the Eaton Endowment Fund. Perhaps this change in status was provoked by the arrival in the Department of Medicine of a cheque for $1,000,000 from the Mead Johnson Company as a contribution to the division of paediatrics for the phenomenally successful baby food, Pablum ™, it had developed. The cheque, made out to the Department of Medicine, had to be endorsed by Duncan Graham before it could be handed over to Dr. Fred Tisdall of the Hospital for Sick Children.

In spite of the generous endowment by the Eaton Endowment Fund, the Department of Medicine was not immune to the harsh impact of the Great Depression of the 1930s. The University Department enjoyed relatively stable financing, but the Hospital fared much worse.

The Hospital's problems were highlighted in the 1935 and 1936 Annual Reports of the Chairman of the Board of Trustees, Mr. Mark Irish. Irish was much concerned over the chronic problem of vacant beds in the Private Pavilion, the revenue from which was needed to support the public wards. He stated:

> Investigations would lead us to believe that our difficulty lies in our relationship with the University, the details of which ... are fairly well understood by all of you, but its main feature is the appointment of our Medical Staff through the Department of Medicine of the University, and the teaching feature thereby implied ... The Chairman of the Medical Advisory Board [Dr. Duncan Graham] had no hesitancy in expressing to me the opinion that his duties, and the duties of his colleagues, are [the] rearing of great doctors, and, as soon as they have reached greatness, passing them out to other institutions, and beginning over again with raw material.[11]

There can be little doubt that Irish's remarks were directed primarily at Duncan Graham whose private practice had remained small, contributing little to the hospital's finances that were largely dependent on occupancy of beds in the Private Pavilion.

Irish's plea was one that has been repeated by many directors of teaching hospitals in times of financial stress. Either the hospital must be opened to "all medical practitioners of registered standing," Irish said, "or we must ask the University to contribute toward the operating deficits."

He concluded his 1936 Annual Report saying:

> To the Medical Advisory Board, and to the services under it, I tender my thanks. According to their lights, which at times I may have thought burned dimly, I believe the doctors have treated me with consideration. From my experience, however, I refrain from reflecting that, affili-

ated as we are with the University, the success of its Medical Department is wrapped up in the success of this Hospital...I have been quite unable to convey to the medical faculty that revenue from the Private Patients' Pavilion is absolutely essential to the maintenance of the public wards.[12]

Irish wanted to see the medical staff augmented from 125 to 200 so as to fill the empty beds on the private wards. It was rumoured that, because Duncan Graham had so few patients in the private wards, he should be replaced by Dr. Herbert K. Detweiler, who had a large private practice. Detweiler is said to have refused to consider such a course. At an emergency Sunday meeting of the Department from which Graham was absent, he joined in a unanimous vote that, if Duncan Graham were asked to resign, the entire staff would submit their resignations.

We do not know what effect this vote of confidence had on the Board of Trustees, although the succeeding Chairman, Mr. E.C. Fox, initiated no further action and the *status quo* was maintained. Perhaps this was because the medical service at the Toronto Western Hospital was reorganized shortly afterwards with Dr. Detweiler as Physician-in-Chief. Certainly the changes proposed by Irish would have seriously impaired the Department's teaching program.

As it was, during Graham's tenure as department head, some 130 physicians underwent graduate training in internal medicine or one of its subspecialties. Of these, many went on to academic positions, either at Toronto, elsewhere in Canada, or in the United States. Five became department chairmen, thus extending Graham's influence to medical schools across the country. The Department also provided training opportunities for many physicians on their way to specialization in surgery, radiology and paediatrics.[13]

Graham insisted on his right to review and approve every paper submitted for publication from his department. This annoyed some staff members who resented what they saw as an unnecessary delay. Unlike many department heads of the day, he never put his name to a paper unless he had been directly involved in the work.

One rather crude measure of the department's growth and influence under Graham can be found in the number of publications in learned journals by members of the staff. In 1919-20, the year of his appointment, there were 20. By 1938-39, the last pre-war year, this had risen to 40.[14] There were significant studies of Simmonds' disease and hypoparathyroid tetany by R. F. Farquharson; work on the production

Sir John Eaton.

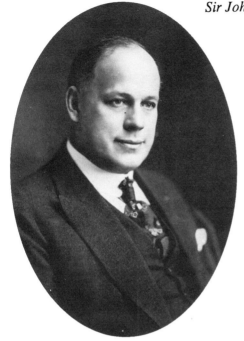

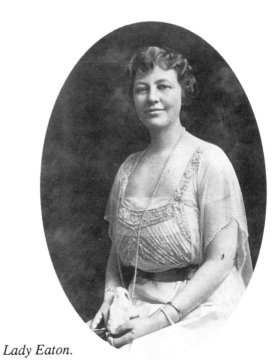

Lady Eaton.

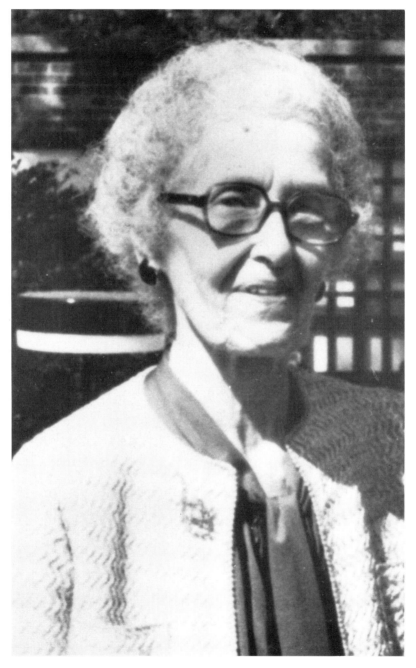

*Miss Stella Clutton, Secretary for the Department of Medicine,
1922-61.*

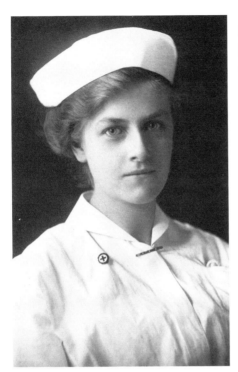

*Enid Gordon Finley
(Mrs Duncan Graham),
1917.*

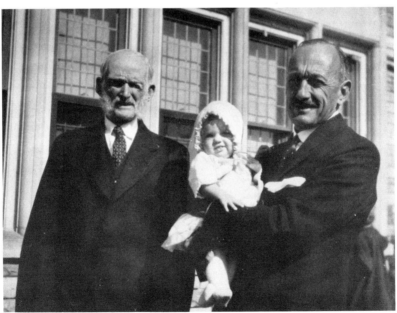

Graham's father (left) and Graham with daughter Enid Mary.

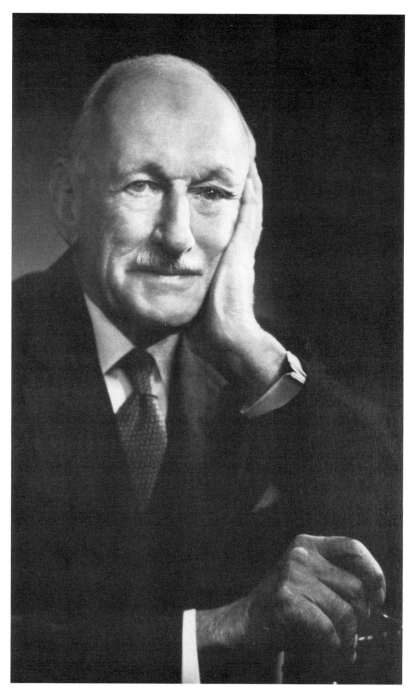

Duncan A.L. Graham in later years.

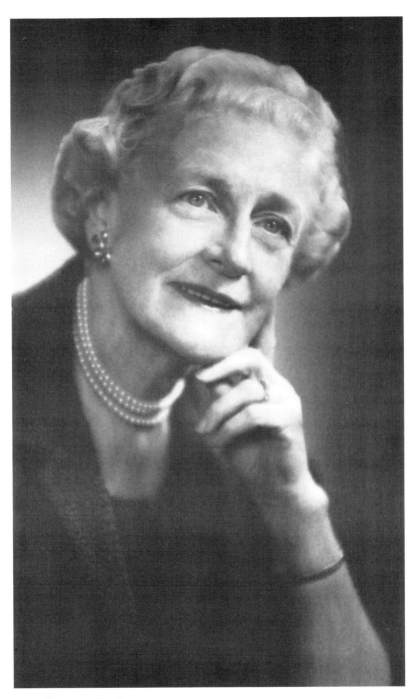

Mrs. Duncan Graham.

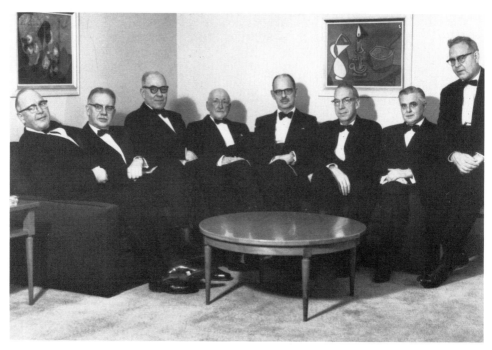

Graham's 80th birthday, January 8, 1962. Heads of Department of medicine whose training was under DG, from left to right, R.C. Dickson (Dalhousie), Dr. W.F. Connell (Queen's), Dr. R.F. Farquharson (Toronto), DG, Dr. K.J.R. Wightman (Toronto), Dr. I.M. Hilliard (Saskatchewan), Dr. R.B. Kerr (British Columbia) (co-author), Dr. F.S. Brien (Western Ontario).

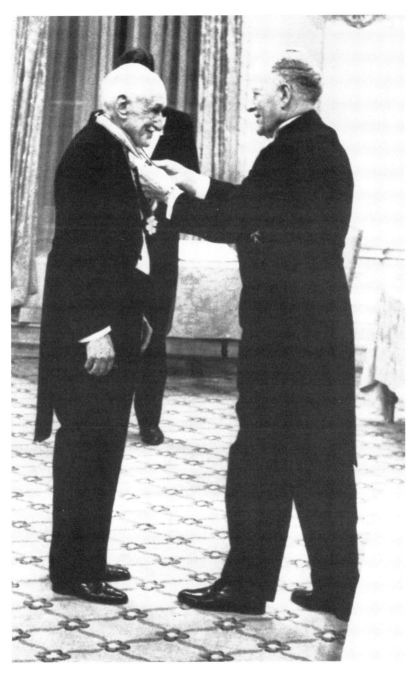

Investiture as Companion of the Order of Canada by Governor General Roland Michener, Government House, November 12, 1968.

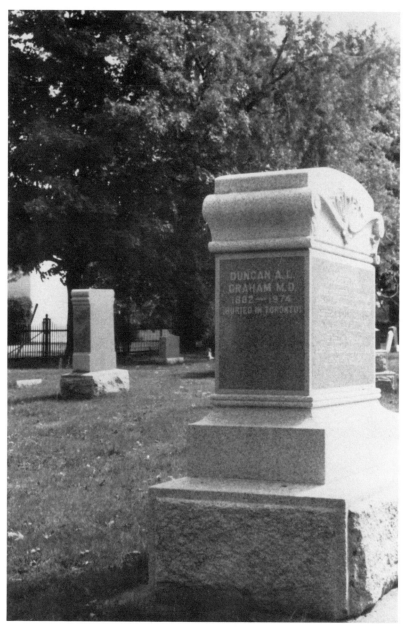

Graham family tombstone, Melville United Church graveyard, Lobo Township, Middlesex County, Ontario. Duncan Graham's ashes are buried in Mount Pleasant Cemetery, Toronto.

of adrenal cortical extract, on adrenal cortical function and the treatment of Addison's disease by R. A. Cleghorn; the use of protamine zinc insulin by W. R. Campbell and A. A. Fletcher, as well as studies of bronchiectasis by W. P. Warner. Farquharson and H. H. Hyland reported studies on the improvement in the neurological complications in pernicious anaemia patients treated with liver extract. Graham's own researches covered a wide spectrum that included tuberculosis and other infectious diseases, the iodine treatment of goitre, various anaemias, nephritis, jaundice, arthritis, endocrine disease and peripheral vascular disorders. In 1923, he was an invited contributor to the *Nelson Loose Leaf Medicine* and, two decades later, to the equally distinguished *Oxford Loose Leaf System of Medicine*.[15]

By the time Duncan Graham stepped down as its Chairman in 1947, the Department of Medicine at the University of Toronto was firmly established as one of the outstanding departments in North America. While this cannot be taken as a single-handed accomplishment of Graham, it is clear that his was the pivotal role in the evolution of what became, as it has remained, a renowned department.

CHAPTER XI
MARRIAGE AND FAMILY

In the years immediately following World War I the importance of rehabilitation began to be appreciated at many of Canada's larger, more forward-looking hospitals. The stimulus for this interest doubtless came largely from the experience of those concerned with the restoration to the work force of the more severely disabled military veterans who were being cared for in the country's veterans' hospitals.

At the time, physiotherapy was the principal means used for the restoration of the disabled. One of its early practitioners was a young Montreal woman, Enid Gordon Finley, the daughter of a well-to-do Montreal family. Enid had spent the final three years of her schooling in Europe, two of them in Geneva and one in Heidelberg. Following this she had studied physiotherapy in Philadelphia, returning to Montreal to teach in McGill's School of Physical Education.[1]

Toward the end of the war she moved to Toronto and became Supervising Masseuse at an institution with the delightfully archaic name — The Hart House School of Massage and Orthopaedic Surgery. The school had been established to train physiotherapists for the country's military hospitals. A short time later she married Dr. L. Bruce Robertson, a young surgeon on the staff of the Hospital for Sick Children. Robertson had served overseas with a Canadian Casualty Clearing Station where he had done pioneering work in the use of blood transfusion for battle casualties.

The few short years of their marriage were busy ones for Enid. In 1920, when Enid was only twenty-four, she persuaded the Medical Advisory Board of the Toronto General Hospital to authorize the establishment in the hospital wards of a course of instruction in remedial gymnastics, one of the names by which physiotherapy was then known. The one-man committee that had been appointed by the Medical Advisory Board to consider Mrs. Robertson's proposal was the Professor of Medicine, Duncan Graham.[2] After she had drawn up a detailed plan, doubtless in consultation with Dr. Graham, her proposal was approved. Two years later, in 1922, the promising career of Dr. Robertson was tragically cut short by his death at the age of thirty-eight. The young widow now had two small children to cope with, Lorraine and Alan.

While still in her widow's weeds, Mrs. Robertson arrived at Graham's office, looking for the office of the Toronto Academy of Medicine, to which she wanted to donate her late husband's medical books. Duncan gallantly took her in tow and guided her to the Academy offices. On his return he remarked to Stella Clutton on the young widow's remarkable attractiveness.

Not long after, Enid packed up her two children and left for Europe where she spent the next three years, travelling and visiting friends in Switzerland, Italy and Britain. The children were occasionally parked with friends while Enid went off on ski-trips or mountain climbing. When the youngsters were approaching school age she decided that she should bring them back to Toronto. There she immediately immersed herself in the promotion of a university School of Physiotherapy. She was joined in this by Miss Kathleen McMurrich. Their efforts were finally rewarded when the University of Toronto School of Physiotherapy was opened in 1929.[3]

During this period she met Duncan Graham frequently at social gatherings of mutual friends. It was obvious that he shared her interest in the School, and, as it turned out, in other things as well. The couple was quietly married at a simple ceremony at St. Andrew's Presbyterian Church on June 20th, 1929. After a honeymoon of two months in British Columbia and Europe, they returned to Toronto to a house they had bought on Spadina Road.

One cannot help wondering at the magnitude of the adjustment that each of the newlyweds had to make. He was a bachelor of 47 who had been living in an apartment close to hospital where he had been tended by a Chinese manservant. She was a 33-year-old widow of some means with two children. She was widely travelled, independent, and had experienced the excitement of personal accomplishment. The two strong personalities clearly found what they sought in each other. The marriage lasted forty-five serene years until Mrs. Graham's death.

Graham's medical colleagues, students and residents detected a decided mellowing in his temperament after his marriage. The Graham house became noted for its frequent graceful dinner parties. The Grahams were also regular hosts of the evening meetings of the Toronto Branch of the Alpha Omega Alpha Honor Medical Society, of which Graham was a Counselor. At parties and in receiving lines, Mrs. Graham would stand at Graham's side quietly whispering to him the names of guests as they stepped forward to be welcomed. Many credited Duncan with a remarkable memory that, by right, was his wife's.

On April 23, 1930, Mrs. Graham gave birth to a daughter, Enid Mary. The next day Dr. Graham was greeted by a standing ovation from his class when he entered the lecture theatre.

Life in the Graham household was well-ordered and generally tranquil. The children, Alan and Lorraine, got on well with their new step-father and he with them, and all of them with the new baby, Enid Mary. Alan remembers his stepfather as being even-handed in his treatment of the children, all being welcome, but none favoured over the others. At home, as in his professional life, Duncan Graham was taciturn and reserved. He was not given to praise and family members came to recognize that his silent twinkle was a high compliment. Graham took pains to avoid undue influence over the children in their plans for adult life. Alan particularly remembers how careful he was not to push him toward the medical career he eventually chose.

The family spent their summer vacations at their cottage, Pine Ridge, at Sturgeon Lake where Mrs. Graham put all her effort into the flower garden while Dr. Graham "managed the compost heap." Alan describes his stepfather as having been "handy" about the house and cottage, though not the kind of do-it-yourselfer who engages in intricate construction projects. He was, however, a capable and canny supervisor of the workmen the couple engaged for these projects.

One of Graham's favourite relaxations during the summer months was golf. He played a good game and he played it with gusto, if not quite the skill of a champion. He was also a keen fly-fisherman, a pastime he pursued at the Caledon Club, a private trout club north of Toronto. For less strenuous relaxation he played bridge, meeting regularly at the York Club with Drs. William Goldie and John Oille.

Enid Mary grew up to marry Dr. John M. Lewis with whom she had six children. She is now Mrs L. N. Hogarth and lives in Bracebridge, Ontario. She recalls a pact that was entered into by her parents. Duncan was not enthusiastic about dancing but Mrs. Graham very much enjoyed it. She was also a devotee of mountain climbing, a sport she had come to love during her years in Switzerland. She persuaded Duncan that she would give up dancing if he would take up mountain climbing. Why Graham agreed to forsake the safety of ballroom dancing for the danger of mountaineering has never been revealed. He must have thought she was worth it! Anyway, he threw himself into the new venture. The couple became members of the Alpine Club and went to the Rockies almost every summer to climb. Duncan achieved the highest qualification in the sport. As soon as they were old enough, the children were taken on mountain climbing expeditions. All of them, and most of the grandchildren, became, and have remained, enthusiastic climbers.

In their later years, when mountaineering became too risky, Duncan relented and joined his wife in dancing lessons at the Arthur Murray Dance Studio. In time they became sufficiently expert to help organize the dances for the 48th Highlanders' annual Burns Night.

CHAPTER XII
DUNCAN GRAHAM AND THE ROYAL COLLEGE

During the nineteen-twenties there was a growing desire in Canadian medicine that doctors who had achieved distinction and who restricted their professional activities to a particular kind of practice should receive formal recognition. A handful of physicians had undertaken extended postgraduate training in Britain and had returned to Canada as Members or Fellows of one of the Royal Colleges of Physicians or Surgeons of England, Edinburgh or Dublin. They were quickly recognized as leaders in the profession and many of them rose rapidly to senior ranks in the country's medical schools.

Certain of these men (there were no women) believed that Canada should establish a Royal College or Colleges patterned on, or affiliated with the British Colleges. Others, particularly among the surgeons, favoured establishing formal connection with the American colleges of physicians and surgeons. Among Quebec francophones, the sentiment leaned toward affiliation with specialty societies in France. These disparate views were promoted and debated at meetings of the Canadian Medical Association and at the more recently formed (1912) Medical Council of Canada.[1] Difficulties in harmonizing these divergent opinions kept the debate going throughout the twenties, and little real progress was made. It was only toward the end of the decade that a consensus began to emerge in favour of forming what was to become the Royal College of Physicians and Surgeons of Canada.

At the time, Canada's population was only about ten million. There were fewer than nine thousand physicians, compared to more than forty thousand today, and the country's nine medical schools were graduating an annual average of 450 new doctors, compared with the current output of more than 1,700 from sixteen schools.

In the twenties, the academic doctors of medical faculties played an even larger role in directing the health care system than they do now. If we assume no more than a hundred physicians per faculty (it may have been fewer), then it can be inferred that the destiny of the nation's health was decided by a small proportion of the medical academics who numbered no more than eight hundred. Duncan Graham was one of the most prominent of this élite.

Although Graham himself does not appear to have been active in the twenties in promoting the formation of the Royal College, one of his Toronto surgical colleagues, F. N. G. Starr, had been pressing for it at the CMA as early as 1913. Starr was joined in his advocacy by a fellow Toronto surgeon, Alexander Primrose, who had served with Graham in Salonika and who became Dean of the medical faculty in 1920.[2] Both Starr and Primrose were members of the CMA's Nucleus Committee which, under the chairmanship of CMA President, Dr. David Low of Regina, worked between 1927 and 1929 to develop the proposal that led to the formation of the College in 1929. Since Graham's talents as an organizer and planner were now well established and widely recognized, he must have been prominent among the Toronto faculty members whom Starr and Primrose consulted.

The proposal of the Nucleus Committee gave special recognition to physicians "who have achieved distinction in some branch of the medical profession as evidenced by their holding professorships in recognized Canadian Medical Schools or displaying high ability in one or more special departments of the medical profession...".[3] Thus a sort of club of medical academics with specialized interests was proposed. Admission to the club was to be by examination. It was only later that the College assumed the role of certifying *all* specialists.

The skillful sponsorship of Dr. A. MacGillivray Young of Saskatoon, a member of CMA's Executive Committee and a Member of Parliament, with other physician-parliamentarians, ensured the passage of an Act to incorporate the Royal College of Physicians and Surgeons of Canada. Royal Assent was given on June 14, 1929.[4]

In November 1929, seventy-two men, including Graham, met in Ottawa as the Provisional Council of the new College. The main function was to establish a permanent structure to carry on the affairs of the College. This newly constituted Council was to consist of eighteen members, two from each medical school, one physician and one surgeon. Starr and Graham were chosen from Toronto. When it came to the election of officers, Graham proposed that, in addition to the President, there should be two Vice-Presidents, one for surgery and one for medicine. His suggestion was adopted and Jonathan C. Meakins of McGill was named President, with Starr and Graham as the Vice-Presidents. This organizational structure for the Officers of the College has been continued to the present day.

Meakins was succeeded as President by Starr in 1931, and in 1933 Duncan Graham became President. During his eight years as a member of the Council of the College Graham was a member of the important Committee on Fellowship, Credentials and Examinations. It was this Committee that established the criteria for the admission of Charter Fellows, and set up the rules and regulations governing the examinations for the admission of others to Fellowship. The Committee elected to have two examinations, following the pattern of the English Royal College — a primary examination in the basic sciences and a final, clinical examination.

Meakins and Graham were named as the Board of Examiners for the College's first final examinations in medicine. They were to continue as the medical Board of Examiners for the next thirteen years. The first final examinations in surgery were held in 1932 and those in medicine three years later. After the 1932 examinations, the surgical candidates were ushered into a room to confront the gowned examiners, one of whom greeted them with, "Gentlemen, you were not good enough. Good afternoon." The first candidates in medicine, in 1935, fared no better. The next year two medical candidates, both of whom passed, were Dr. J.A. Dauphinee of Toronto and Dr. J. E. Plunkett of Ottawa.

At first the College's annual meetings were devoted only to business and social activities. However, by 1932 attendance, almost entirely from Quebec and Ontario, had fallen sharply and it was decided that a scientific program was needed if more were to be attracted to future meetings. Duncan Graham was named chairman of a small committee and the first scientific program was presented the following year. Wilder Penfield and John Beattie of McGill and R.I. Harris of Toronto were the speakers. Graham and his committee recruited speakers of comparable distinction for subsequent meetings and, by 1939, attendance had more than doubled and cross-country representation had broadened.[5]

Although the need for a standard of qualification for specialists had been discussed at many levels during the 1920s, only Alberta gave the idea legal recognition, based on certificates issued by the Registrar of the University of Alberta.[6] In Ontario, advocacy for specialty standards other than Fellowship of the Royal College led E. Stanley Ryerson, secretary to Toronto's Medical Faculty, to make other proposals. In a 1933 editorial in the *Canadian Medical Association Journal*, Ryerson suggested that qualifications for the recognition of specialists be established by the Medical Council of Canada, which was already in the business of conducting examinations accepted by the provinces as a basis for general medical licensure.[7]

The response to Ryerson's editorial was a comic opera of sluggish and reluctant buck passing that went on for the next three years. Ryerson, with good reason, had been fearful that unless action were taken by some central body provinces were likely to set up independent and varied standards for specialty qualification. He advocated circumventing such an unwelcome development through the establishment of centrally administered certificates of competence to be awarded to those whose educational attainments were midway between those of the Medical Council of Canada and those of Royal College Fellowship.

J. Fenton Argue, Registrar of the Medical Council, seems not to have been enthusiastic over the proposal and did not pursue it with any vigour. A frustrated Ryerson then lobbied the Executive Committee of the CMA, which responded in 1934 by naming him chairman of a committee to study the question. By this time Duncan Graham was President of the Royal College and also a member of Ryerson's committee.

Up to this point the College had not been involved in the discussions of specialist certification. However, at Graham's behest, it now decided it should look into the matter and appointed a committee under J. G. Fitzgerald to represent the College. The College and CMA committees met in joint session in October 1934. The College was poorly represented at the meeting and took no action. The CMA, however, again endorsed the Medical Council as the body that should be responsible for the certification of specialists.

When Ryerson approached the Medical Council again in October 1935, he was rebuffed by its opinion that specialist certification was outside the powers of the Medical Council as laid down in the Canada Medical Act. The next month Duncan Graham reported to the Royal College's Annual Meeting that the College was now considering granting diplomas in certain medical and surgical specialties. The incoming College President, A.T. Bazin of Montreal, then appointed Graham chairman of the Committee on Specialists. Graham's committee felt it could not act until the Medical Council formally withdrew its candidacy as a specialist certifying body, which it did in September 1936.[8]

Writing about this period in *The Royal College of Surgeons of Canada: 1920-1960*, Sclater Lewis says, "He [Graham] was firmly convinced of the future success of the College, but felt that it could only fulfil its function by maintaining high standards, not only in its requirements of postgraduate training but also in the quality of its examinations. His services and advice were of the greatest value when the College undertook the task of specialist certification."[9]

Meanwhile, the Canadian Association of Radiologists, exasperated at the delays, threatened to proceed independently with the establishment of a College of Radiology. In a typical manifestation of Canadian *politesse*, the College decided it should not act until formally invited to do so by the Canadian Medical Association. This invitation was not forthcoming until a year later, in October 1937, when an official invitation to the Royal College to assume responsibility for the certification of specialists was issued from CMA's Annual Meeting.

While awaiting action by the CMA Graham's committee was not idle. Recognizing that the College ought to say why it should be in the business of certifying specialists, the committee set about preparing such a statement. It also identified the specialties it regarded as suitable for certification, and the general principles to be followed when laying down training requirements that candidates in each specialty should meet. The College was thus well prepared when the invitation finally came. The committee's report became the basis for the relatively uniform standards for specialist certification that were eventually adopted.

Meanwhile, Graham was somehow able to placate the radiologists, as well as the ophthalmologists, otolaryngologists and anaesthetists, all of whom were now restive, insistent on action and threatening to form independent certifying bodies. Records of the Royal College Council meetings make it clear that, but for the patient efforts and negotiating skills of Duncan Graham, specialist certification in Canada would most likely have evolved as a cluster of independent, poorly coordinated, small specialty colleges. James H. Graham (no relation), the College's long-time Secretary, has said, "There is no doubt that Duncan Graham was the real father of the certification program." The unique strength of Canada's Royal College is that it encompasses all specialty certification under a single tightly coordinated agency in a way that has been accomplished in only one other country — South Africa.[10]

With remarkable prescience Graham had advised the Council of the Royal College in 1935 that, "Should we have some form of health insurance in Canada, it is quite evident that there will be a sharp division between what is known as general practice and what is known as special practice. If we had some simple method of classifying specialists we could appeal to the governments requesting them to consider as specialists those doctors holding diplomas of this College."[11]

CHAPTER XIII
WORLD WAR II AND THE PROFESSOR'S MANY HATS

The small size of Canada's medical establishment in the 1920s and 30s made it inevitable that the reins of power would be in the hands of an élite. It was also inevitable that this élite would function as a sort of Old Boy's network to facilitate the passing back and forth of the high offices in the major national organizations. Thus it was that between 1927 and 1951 the presidency of the Canadian Medical Association was six times held by individuals who either had been, or would be, presidents of the Royal College of Physicians and Surgeons.

The interlock between the two most powerful national medical bodies of the day began with F. N. G. Starr, who became President of the CMA in 1927-28 and of the Royal College in 1931-33. J.C. Meakins, the Royal College's first President (1929-31) became President of the CMA in 1935-36. A.T. Bazin was CMA President in 1929-30 and Royal College President from 1935 to 1937. The sequence was reversed in Duncan Graham's case. He had been Royal College President from 1933 to 1935 and went on to the CMA presidency in the war years of 1940-41. F. S. Patch, who was CMA President in 1939-40, became Royal College President in 1943-45. The 1943-44 CMA President, D. Sclater Lewis of Montreal, assumed the Royal College presidency in 1949-51.[1]

This overlapping of the executive officers of the two bodies was vitally important to the fledgling Royal College whose existence and role had to have the approval and support of the main body of the profession, which was represented by the CMA. In more recent years, overlap in the interests of the two organizations has diminished as the interests of each have diverged. The Royal College, like other specialized bodies spawned by the CMA, grew in size and strength to the point where it could maintain itself without the support of its parent.

Duncan Graham, at 57, was at the peak of his powers at the outbreak of World War II in 1939. It was only natural that, after the initial social chaos that follows the declaration of any war, his help would be sought in defining and implementing the role of the Canadian medical profession.

Almost immediately, he was appointed as consulting physician on the staff of the Director General of Medical Services of the Canadian Army with the rank of Colonel. The appointment did not require him to give up his position as Professor of Medicine at the University of Toronto, or Physician-in-Chief at the Toronto General Hospital, since both institutions agreed to his spending two days a week in Ottawa with the Director General, Col. R. M. Gorssline. The arrangement was also acceptable to the Canadian Medical Association, of which he became President-elect in early 1940.[2]

The added responsibilities of these commitments threw a strain not only on Graham, but on his entire department and, indeed, on the University itself. Of the forty-four members of the staff in the Department of Medicine, eighteen would eventually enlist for active service. Two more served part-time and four acted as consultants to the Armed Forces. Wing Commander Ray F. Farquharson became consultant to the Royal Canadian Air Force, and Brigadier W. P. Warner became Deputy Director of Medical Services (Army). In his Annual Report on the Department in 1943 Graham wrote, "Almost all members of the staff of military age and physically fit are on active service."[3]

The burden this placed on the remaining staff was further aggravated in 1942 when the medical course was accelerated by the elimination of summer vacations for both students and professors, so that teaching continued round the clock for twelve months of the year. To help contend with the added load many older physicians postponed their retirement. Research had to be curtailed, and the department's post-graduate program was disrupted through enlistment.

It is doubtful if Graham would have been able to cope with the added burden had not the skillful and effective support of the incomparable Stella Clutton been available to him. Her secretarial responsibilities were now expanded to encompass much of the day-to-day management of the Department. She arranged time-tables, booked classrooms, dragooned professors to their teaching assignments and quietly assumed responsibility for keeping the Department on an even keel. Her only vacation during the war years came on the Labour Day weekend of 1945, after the end of hostilities. Though her efforts were not formally recognized at the time, she was rewarded at her retirement in 1961 with the Sesquicentennial Long Service Award, the citation of which reads, in part: "That Stella Clutton made major contributions to the success of the Department was clearly proven during the Second World War when the heads of the Departments of Medicine and of Therapeutics...served in Ottawa as consultants.... She assumed administrative responsibilities for both departments...."[4]

As a member of the CMA's General Council and Executive Committee, Graham was ideally placed as consultant to the military. He was able to advise both the Army and the Association on the wartime allocation of medical services to meet civilian and military needs. One such need that was particularly pressing was the medical examination of recruits. In discussions between representatives of the Department of National War Services and the CMA it was agreed that examinations could be carried out by any qualified medical practitioner in good standing. Military physicians were thus freed for other duties, while practitioners could attend to their civilian practices when they were not examining recruits. The fee for each examination was $1.00, an amount considered equivalent to the pay of an army Medical Officer.[5]

The Association also agreed to nominate doctors to serve on Medical Boards to re-examine recruits. A Board consisted of a physician, a surgeon and, where available, an eye, ear, nose and throat specialist. Graham met frequently and at length to work out the composition and role of the Boards with Major-General (Ret.) L. R. La Flèche, the Deputy Minister of National Defence.

Under Graham's presidency the CMA established a Central Medical Advisory Committee to link the Divisional Military District Committees that had been established in each Province. They advised District Military, Navy and Air Force Offices on the best ways to assure adequate numbers of medical officers for the armed services, and, so far as possible, for the civilian population. The success of the Committees was highly variable, depending on the local personalities serving on them.

Graham was much concerned over the spotty and haphazard performance of the Divisional Committees. He opened a meeting of the CMA Executive Committee in 1941 saying, "I wonder if we have done our part." He went on to note that in one military district the Divisional Advisory Committee "might as well not exist." In another it was noted that "among the men recommended" (by the District Medical Officer) "...were two who were drunks and of no use to the service."[6]

In September 1942, after two and a half years of service, Graham resigned his commission as Consultant to the DGMS. This was probably necessitated by the demands of his growing list of other commitments and of his department at the University, which by now had reached its most severe state of manpower depletion.

In June 1941 Graham reported to the CMA's Executive Committee that he and Dr. T. H. Leggett, the chairman of CMA's General Council, had learned that the Deputy Minister of Pensions and National Health,

Dr. Wodehouse, had been instructed to develop a plan of health insurance to be submitted to Parliament by the Minister at the forthcoming session of Parliament. After considerable discussion Graham moved that the Executive Committee approve:

> That the Canadian Medical Association is in favour of any plan to make available for every Canadian the full benefits of curative and preventive medicine, irrespective of individual ability to pay, which at the same time, is given at a rate of remuneration which is fair to the public and to the practitioners of medicine and others associated in the provision of medical care, but the Canadian Medical Association is not in favour of State Medicine — 'a system of medical administration by which the state provides medical services for the entire population or a large part thereof and under which all practitioners are employed, directed and paid by the state on a salary basis or otherwise.'
>
> The Canadian Medical Association considers as a necessary requisite for any plan of community medical service adopted, the unification of curative and preventive medicine in medical practice.[7]

Thus, with the country deeply engaged in a prodigious war effort, the Canadian Medical Association, at Duncan Graham's urging, looked a quarter century into the future in adopting a pro-medicare stance.

As an observer and participant in the progress of medical science, Graham was aware of the beginnings of the explosion in medical knowledge that was to characterize the decade of the forties and beyond. In his view this made it a matter of urgency for the CMA to prepare itself for increased government participation in the provision of the benefits of medical advances to the public. The CMA's Committee on Economics had made extensive studies of the economics of health insurance plans in place in other countries, and Graham strongly endorsed the view that the problem of providing medical services could not be solved in Canada by a system of State Medicine in which Doctors became state employees. A solution could only be found, he said in his valedictory address as CMA President, "through a cooperative effort on the part of the organized medical profession, government, public welfare organizations, and the public."[8]

He went on to say:

> It remains our first duty and responsibility as an Associa-
> tion to ensure that the medical care provided will be of a
> high standard which will be maintained and strengthened
> as medical knowledge advances. If medical service is to be
> rendered in accordance with the honorable traditions of
> our profession and its code of ethics, and the four funda-
> mental conditions necessary for an efficient medical serv-
> ice fulfilled, namely: intelligent application of existing
> knowledge, unification of curative and preventive medi-
> cine; division and acceptance of responsibilities among
> those in general and special practice; and recognition of
> the hospital as the chief center of specialist medical serv-
> ice, then medical care must begin in the home, embrace the
> curative and preventive aspects of medicine, and be under
> the direction of a general practitioner with the necessary
> training and qualifications.

He then challenged the Association. "Is, then, the medical profession going to permit its rightful functions to be usurped by governments
in response to the growing demand of the public for a more adequate
medical service? Or are members of the profession willing to act in this
vital matter as an organized body and give what should be and must be
a cooperative effort, effective guidance and leadership?"[9]

In his meetings with General La Flèche, Graham was much concerned with the recruitment of medical graduates to serve in the armed
forces. To facilitate the recruitment of medical officers he volunteered
the CMA's services in ascertaining the military service intentions of
recent medical graduates during their internships. He insisted, however, that graduates must complete at least one year of internship before
enlisting. He also urged the CMA to make what efforts it could to
ensure that the interests of those physicians who had gone overseas
would be protected when they returned.

It is often said that if you want to get a job done quickly and
efficiently you should find someone who is already overloaded with
work and ask him to do it. Since 1939, Graham's friend, Sir Frederick
Banting, had been chairman of the National Research Council's
Associate Committee on Aviation Research. Graham became the
Committee's vice-chairman in 1940. In 1941 when Banting was killed
on his way to England, Graham succeeded to the the chairmanship of

the Committee. This made him a member *ex-officio* of the subcommittees on Psychology and Personnel Selection, Oxygen Equipment, and Protective Clothing. Graham was also a member of the the National Research Council and of its Associate Committee on Medical Research. In this capacity he served as Chairman of the Subcommittee on Wound Infections and as a member of the Subcommittee on Shock and Blood Substitutes. As if these responsibilities were not enough, he was also a member of the National Research Council's Associate Committee on Army Medical Research.[10]

The many hats that Duncan Graham wore during the war years brought social responsibilities that fell largely on Mrs. Graham. It was she who had to arrange the spouses' programs at CMA meetings and see to it that the important social side of the meetings went smoothly. She also saw to the entertaining of Duncan's various committees when they met in Toronto with small receptions and dinner parties. In addition, Mrs. Graham continued to be active in the affairs of the Canadian Physiotherapy Association of which she had been a co-founder. She set up the Association's Military Affairs Committee which was concerned with recruitment of Association members into the armed forces. This Committee was instrumental in gaining the status of officer rank for physiotherapists in military service.

The Grahams' family life during the war years was a busy whirl with little time for treasured evenings at home. Somehow they managed to hold things together; the marriage seems even to have strengthened under the pressures of a multitude of extraneous forces.

CHAPTER XIV
EASING UP

In 1947, after 28 years as Professor and Head of the Department of Medicine, Duncan Graham reached the mandatory retirement age of 65. The occasion was marked, as such occasions almost always are, by a formal dinner put on by past and present staff members at Toronto's distinguished York Club. Dr. John Hepburn, one of Graham's early protégés, was the toastmaster and Dean J. A. MacFarlane joined the redoubtable William Goldie and Walter R. Campbell in tributes to Dr. Graham. In a gracious response Graham warned his colleagues that medicine was not just a single service but encompassed the application of knowledge from all branches of medicine to diagnosis and treatment. The presentation portrait by Lillias Newton vividly depicts Graham in his academic robes, looking directly at the viewer with an intent and quizzical eye.

Other tributes quickly followed. The University appointed him Professor Emeritus and awarded him the Honorary Degree of LL.D. Other honorary degrees were conferred by the University of Western Ontario and Queen's University. In each case the citation emphasized Graham's honesty, integrity and dedication to the highest standards in his students and professional colleagues. In this spate of adulation it is clear that Graham's peers saw him as an outstanding example for students and practitioners.[1]

Among the many other honours and awards that came to him were the Canadian Medical Association's highest award, the F. N. G. Starr Award, which is given for outstanding contribution to science, the fine arts or literature, service to humanity or improvement of medical services. He was also made Honorary Fellow of the Royal College of Physicians of London, Fellow of the Royal Society of Canada, Fellow of the American College of Physicians, member of the Association of American Physicians and the American Society of Clinical Investigation. In 1944 he was made Commander of the Order of the British Empire. He had received the Coronation Medal in 1937 and was given the Confederation Medal in 1967. The American College of Physicians gave him its Distinguished Teacher Award and, in 1968, he joined the select company of Companions of the Order of Canada.

Like many who are required to drop the reins of responsibility at an age when their capabilities and zest are undiminished, Duncan Graham refused to go peacefully into a retirement of total leisure. He kept his nose in his former department to an extent that some thought was excessive. He spent a good deal of time in the department library where he continued writing. John D. Hamilton, who was then Dean of the Faculty, tells that Graham came to him several times to criticize the direction in which the department was being moved by his successors, R. F. Farquharson and, later, K. J. R. Wightman. He was particularly critical of the decentralization of teaching away from the Toronto General to other hospitals, a move that was a necessary prelude to the planned enlargement of the medical class. Graham found this too great a deviation from the principle he had established of close and tight central control by the Professor and Head. He also thought that his successors were too heavily engaged in private practice, contrary to the intent of the Eaton endowment. Hamilton, who was firmly committed to the decision to enlarge the medical classes, felt that Graham's reaction was simply a reflection of his own strong personality and his abiding dedication to the principle of firm control by the professor. After more than thirty years, Graham remained committed to the terms under which he had originally assumed the chair.[2]

One post-retirement activity that occupied a good deal of the Professor's time entailed his appointment as Advisor on Medical Education and Research to the Director General of Treatment Services of the Department of Veterans' Affairs. In this capacity he made frequent visits to the Veterans' Affairs hospitals that had been established at major centres from Halifax to Vancouver. He effectively promoted the Department's policy of establishing in the veterans' hospitals residency training programs of a quality that would meet the accreditation standards of the Royal College of Physicians and Surgeons. In urging the requirement that medical staff appointments in veterans' hospitals be approved by the head of the relevant university department he sought to ensure that staff was of university calibre. His concern here was to make sure that the medical care provided to veterans was of top quality and that it contributed to undergraduate and post-graduate medical education.[3]

Although his involvement in medical affairs inevitably diminished with his years of retirement, Graham never permitted himself, nor was he permitted by others, to lapse into complete professional idleness. Both he and Mrs. Graham continued to keep in close touch with his "boys" and their wives. He continued to attend the annual meetings of the Royal College where, invariably, groups of his former trainees would organize a table with the Grahams at the formal banquets. On these occasions his former students found that the austere "Prof" had mellowed. "Dunc" was likely now to show his amusement, not with the customary twinkle of the eyes, but with bursts of laughter that were loud and uncontrolled guffaws.[4]

By the middle 1950s what might be termed the Graham gospel of medical education had spread beyond Toronto to virtually all the English-speaking Canadian medical schools. The departments of medicine at five of the twelve schools were headed by graduates of Graham's Toronto training program, and other graduates were to be found in every department across the land.

In 1956 the five department heads, R. C. Dickson of Dalhousie, Ray F. Farquharson of Toronto, Frank S. Brien of Western Ontario, Irwin Hilliard of Saskatchewan and Robert B. Kerr of British Columbia gathered at Toronto's York Club for a birthday dinner with "The Professor." Six years later his friends celebrated his eightieth birthday at a dinner at Toronto's Royal York Hotel. Guests on that occasion included Mrs. Graham and her son and daughter, Dr. Alan Bruce-Robertson and Mrs. F. L. Hovey, and the Grahams' daughter, Enid Mary — Mrs. John M. Lewis.[5]

In Canada's Centennial Year of 1967 Graham, now eighty-five, presented a mace that had been designed for the Canadian Medical Association, at the Association's Annual Meeting. It was at about this time that his personal physician, Dr. Ian MacDonald, "took his courage in his hands" and advised The Professor that he should abandon his life-long habit of cigarette smoking. Graham accepted the advice in good humour and never smoked again.[6]

Shortly before Graham's death, when he was enfeebled and in a wheelchair, he attended the CMA's 1973 annual meeting in Toronto and joined with the Association's other most senior Past President, Dr. Gordon Fahrni of Vancouver, in strenuous opposition to a motion to discontinue the scientific portion of the Annual Meeting. Vigorous applause greeted the motion's withdrawal.[7]

One of Graham's greatest admirers was his former student, Robert C. Dickson of Dalhousie University. In 1969, Dickson, having solicited contributions to an Educational Fund for the Royal College, persuaded the College to establish the Duncan Graham Award for "distinguished service and contribution in the field of medical education." At the College's 1969 Annual Meeting in Edmonton Graham, now 87, presented the first award to John P. Hubbard, chairman of the National

Board of Medical Examiners of Philadelphia. It is doubtful whether any of the many honours bestowed on Duncan Graham during the years of his retirement touched him more deeply than did this recognition of his efforts in medical education. He later wrote: "I could receive no greater honour than to have my name associated with an award for distinguished service and contribution in the field of medical education and especially an award of the Royal College, initiated and supported by a number of my former pupils and graduate students — Fellows of the College."[8]

In his later retirement years the Grahams spent much time at their cottage, Pine Ridge, situated on an eight hectare site on the east arm of Sturgeon Lake, Ontario, near Sturgeon Point, halfway between Bobcaygeon and Fenelon Falls. Graham cared as conscientiously for his vegetable garden as he had for his university department while Mrs. Graham gave just as tender care to the flower garden. She became known as "The Flower Lady" at nearby Providence United Church where she regularly brought flowers for the altar.

The Grahams' daughter, Enid Mary, recalls that when Graham was not golfing at the Sturgeon Point Golf Club, he was likely to be found playing croquet on the cottage's beautifully manicured lawn or practising his golf swing.[9]

The quiet happiness of the couple's retirement years ended abruptly in June 1973. With Mrs. Graham at the wheel, they were driving close to their summer cottage when a motorcyclist cut in front of them. In avoiding the cyclist the car left the road and hit a tree. Dr. and Mrs. Graham were taken to the Lindsay General Hospital.

Not long after discharge from the hospital, Mrs. Graham suffered a severe stroke that left her with a right sided paralysis and complete loss of speech. She spent the remaining six months of her life in the Toronto General Hospital, unable to communicate except by hand squeezes. She died quietly on January 22, 1974. Because of Graham's debility, her funeral was held in the Graham home so that he could attend.

Shortly after the accident Dr. Graham became jaundiced. It was diagnosed as obstructive — or "surgical" — jaundice. At operation he was found to have a carcinoma of the ampulla of Vater, the point at which the common bile duct discharges into the duodenum. His surgeon, Dr. Frank Mills, decided that Graham would be unlikely to survive the radical surgery for removal of the tumour and performed instead a by-pass operation which relieved the jaundice.

The bed-ridden Professor remained at home, under round-the-clock nursing care. He stubbornly refused to be hospitalized, saying he preferred to die at home. After his wife's death he seemed to lose interest in life and, on February 18th, less than a month later, he, too, quietly slipped away.

EPILOGUE

The forty years that have passed since Duncan Graham stepped down from the Sir John and Lady Eaton Professorship of Medicine have left his footprints in the sands of time as clear and sharp as when he made them. The Eaton Professorship and the full-time principle that underlies it have become so much a part of medical academic life at the University of Toronto that to question the wisdom of its creation today would be the rankest heresy. The turmoil that surrounded Graham's early days as Professor subsided quickly in the face of his cool, efficient application of the principles of excellence in patient care based on rational education.

The full-time concept that began with Graham's appointment has now become an accepted fact of medical academic life, not only at the University of Toronto, but throughout Canada and the rest of North America. It came about as a result of a timely coalescence of circumstances and personalities that seems providential more than a half-century later, but which was at the time doubtless seen as a logical evolution.

The foresight and dedication to an ideal that led Abraham Flexner to overthrow an outworn and enfeebled system of medical education coincided with the era of successful entrepreneurs. The Eatons and the Flavelles focused their philanthropic concerns on the health and welfare of their less fortunate fellows. Flexner's dream of a revitalized system of medical education became a reality at Toronto when William Goldie, the intermediary, brought Eaton and Flavelle together with Sir Robert Falconer, the University's far-sighted President. That a person of Graham's background and talents was available was due, at least in part, to the stimulus medical research had received from the spectacular advances in laboratory medicine around the turn of the century — advances that excited the imagination of students and young physicians of Graham's vintage. Even so, as Goldie remarked at the time of Graham's retirement, "It is surprising how few candidates there are who meet the standards for a position of that kind. He must be a man of outstanding character, an inspiring teacher, an able organizer, with a thorough grasp of the fundamental sciences."[1]

The emphasis that Graham laid on training in the basic sciences for academic physicians is almost universally accepted in today's world, though the means of its attainment has changed. In Graham's day the only place a young physician could be sure of obtaining a solid grounding in the basic sciences was in one of the basic science departments — anatomy, physiology, bacteriology, pathology or pharmacology. Nowadays, the clinical departments of nearly all medical schools have within them sufficient numbers of well-trained scientists that reliance on basic science departments is no longer always necessary.

One feature of Graham's professorship that we are unlikely to see again is a departmental chairmanship with an incumbency of twenty-eight years. It was this long tenure that made it possible for Graham to mould his department, to train and appoint a strong cadre of staff who shared his views of medical education and research. The Graham influence can be expected to percolate through all of Toronto's Faculty of Medicine for at least the remainder of this century, and possibly much longer.

NOTES

CHAPTER I: *The Child*

1. Historical Atlas, Middlesex County, Ontario, 1878, Lobo Township. Map Division, University of British Columbia Library.
2. Duncan Graham's name is engraved on the family gravestone in the cemetery adjacent to Melville United church (formerly Presbyterian) at the site of the village of Ivan in Lobo Township. His ashes and those of Mrs. Graham are buried in Mount Pleasant Cemetery in Toronto beneath a piece of red rock from Sturgeon Lake, Ontario, near the Graham summer home.
3. J.K. Galbraith, *The Scotch* (Boston: Riverside Press, Houghton Mifflin, 1964).
4. Robert Kelly, husband of Ethel Margaret, daughter of Duncan's brother, David Alexander Graham, personal communication to RBK.

CHAPTER II: *The Young Man*

1. Michael Bliss, *Banting: A Biography* (Toronto: McClelland and Stewart, 1944), 28.
2. University of Toronto Archives, Faculty of Medicine Calendars, 1902-05.
3. Dr. Elizabeth Bagshaw, personal communication to RBK.
4. Duncan Graham. See publications list in Appendix B.
5. Ibid.

CHAPTER III: *Soldier-Scientist*

1. A.R.M. Lower, *Colony to Nation: A History of Canada* (Toronto: McClelland and Stewart, 1978), 459.
2. Margaret McIntosh, personal communication to RBK. Mrs. McIntosh had been a nursing sister at No. 2. Can. Gen. Hosp. at le Tréport, France, 1915.
3. B.H. Liddell Hart, "Salonika Campaigns 1915-18," *Encyclopaedia Britannica* (Chicago et al: 1951), 19: 892.
4. Ibid., 892.
5. War Diary, No. 4 Can. Gen. Hosp., 31 Dec. 1915; and "Number 4 Canadian Hospital — the Letters of Professor J. J. Mackenzie from the Salonika Front" (Toronto: Macmillan, 1933), 44, 63.
6. J.J. Mackenzie, op. cit, 35.
7. War Diary, op. cit., 6 Dec. 1915; 9 Dec. 1915 Mackenzie, op. cit, 73.
8. War Diary, op. cit., 26 Oct. 1916.
9. War Diary, op. cit., 26 Jan. 1916, 9 Feb. 1916; 22 March 1916; 19 April 1916; 5 July 1916.
10. Duncan Graham: "Some Points in the Diagnosis and Treatment of Dysentery occurring in the British Salonika Force," *Lancet*, 1918, 1:51-5; editorial, *Lancet*, op. cit, 67.
11. Kenneth M. Ludmerer, *Learning to Heal* (New York: Basic Books, 1985), ch. 6, "The Birth of Academic Medicine," 123 et seq.
12. Stella Clutton, Personal Communication to RBK.
13. War Diary, op. cit., 7 Jan. 1916.
14. Statement of Service and Qualifications, Lieut. Col. Duncan Archibald Graham, Mentioned in Dispatches, L.G. No. 39404, dated 25-10-17.
15. Col. W.B. Hendry, Letter to C. K. Clarke, 13 Oct. 1917, Correspondence File, No. 4 Can. Gen. Hosp. Archives, University of Toronto.

CHAPTER IV: *Dr. Goldie: Kingmaker*

1. Kenneth M.Ludmerer, op. cit., 103.
2. Ibid., 184 et seq.
3. Ibid., 167.
4. W.G. Cosbie, *The Toronto General Hospital 1819-1965: A Chronicle* (Toronto: Macmillan, 1975), 121.
5. Ibid., 141-3.
6. Statutes of Ontario, Toronto General Hospital Act, 1911, and by-law respecting Medical Staff of the Hospital.
7. A.B. McKillop, "Sir Robert Alexander Falconer," *The Canadian Encyclopedia*, 2nd ed. (Edmonton: Hurtig, 1988), 2:744.
8. Flora McCrea, *Memory's Wall: The Autobiography of Flora McCrea Eaton* (Toronto: Clarke, Irwin, 1950), 39-41.
9. Sir Robert Falconer, Letter to Sir John Eaton, 2 May 1918. Falconer papers re: Eatons, Archives, University of Toronto.

CHAPTER V: *The Search*

1. William Goldie, letter to Sir John Eaton, 11 Sept. 1918, Archives, University of Toronto.
2. Ibid.
3. Ibid.
4. Ibid.
5. Sir Robert Falconer, letter to Capt. William Goldie, 16 Nov. 1918, Archives, University of Toronto.
6. William Goldie, letter to Sir Robert Falconer, 10 Dec. 1918, Archives, University of Toronto.
7. Sir Robert Falconer, letter to Lt. Col. Duncan Graham, 10 Jan. 1919, Archives, University of Toronto.
8. Duncan Graham, letter to Sir Robert Falconer, 1 March 1918, Archives, University of Toronto.
9. Harvey Cushing, *The Life of Sir William Osler* (Oxford: Oxford University Press, 1940), 2: 646.
10. Sir Willaim Osler, letter to President Ira Remsen, Johns Hopkins University, published in *C.M.A.J.*, 1962, 87: 762-5.
11. K.M. Ludmerer, op. cit., 133.
12. D. Sclater Lewis, *Royal Victoria Hospital, 1887-1947* (Montreal: McGill University Press, 1969), 69-70.

CHAPTER VI: *Clean Sweep by the New Broom*

1. Statutes, Province of Ontario, The Toronto General Hospital Act, 1911 and by-law respecting the Medical Staff of the Hospital.
2. Duncan Graham, Letter to Sir Robert Falconer, 8 Sept. 1919, Archives, University of Toronto.
3. Ibid.
4. University of Toronto, Calendars, 1918-19 and 1920-21.

CHAPTER VII: *A Storm of Protest*

1. Editorial, *Can. J. Med. and Surg.*, June 1923, 3.
2. Ibid., 9-10.
3. *Can. Practitioner Review*, 1920, 45:89-90.

4. Sir Robert Falconer, Letter to Members of the Clinical Staff, Faculty of Medicine, University of Toronto, 19 Oct. 1921, Archives, University of Toronto.

5. *Report: Special Committee to inquire into The Organization and Administration of the University of Toronto*, 1923, 5. Archives, Province of Ontario, Toronto.

6. *Transcript of Hearings, Special Committee to inquire into The Organization and Administration of the University of Toronto*, 1923, Archives, Province of Ontario, Toronto.

7. Ibid.

8. Ibid.

9. *Report of Special Committee*, op. cit., 16-7, 20.

CHAPTER VIII: *The Professor's New Program*

1. University of Toronto, Calendars, 1920-25, Archives, University of Toronto.

2. Duncan Graham, Letter to Sir Robert Falconer, 8 Sept. 1919, Archives, University of Toronto.

3. Transcript, *Special Committee to inquire into The Organization and Administration of the University of Toronto* - 1923, Archives, Province of Ontario, Toronto.

4. Board of Governors, University of Toronto Special Committee concerning the Faculty of Medicine, Minutes, 160-3.

5. Irwin Hilliard, Oral History Tape, Hannah Institute for the History of Medicine.

CHAPTER IX: *Banting and Insulin*

1. Michael Bliss, *The Discovery of Insulin* (Toronto: McClelland and Stewart, 1982).

2. Ben Traven, *The Treasure of Sierra Madre* (New York, Hill and Wang, 1967).

3. J.J.R. Macleod, *History of the Researches Leading to the Discovery of Insulin* (1922) - Letter to Col. Albert Gooderham, Toronto, 20 Sept. 1922. Bull. History of Medicine, 52: 3, 298-312 1978.

4. *Toronto Daily Star*, 14 Jan. 1922.

5. Bliss, *Banting*, op. cit., 79.

6. F.G. Banting, W.R. Campbell, A.A. Fletcher, "Further Clinical Experience with Insulin (Pancreatic Extracts) in the treatment of Diabetes Mellitus," *Brit. Med. J.*, 6 Jan. 1923, 8-12.

7. Editorial, *Brit. Med. J*, 6 Jan. 1923, 32-3.

8. Bliss, *The Dicovery of Insulin; Banting*, op. cit.

9. Bliss, "Collip, James Bertram," *The Canadian Encyclopedia*, 2nd ed., 1:460.

10. Bliss, *Banting*, op. cit., 79.

11. F.G. Banting and C.H. Best, "The Internal Secretion of the Pancreas." *J. Lab. and Med.*, 1922, 7:256-71.

12. Banting, Best, H.B. Collip, W.R. Campbell and A.A. Fletcher, Pancreatic Extracts in the Treatment of Diabetes Mellitus," *Can. Med. Assoc. J.*, 1922, 12:141-6.

13. Bliss, "Banting," op. cit., 94.

14. Ibid., 94-5.

15. Minutes, Board of Trustees, Toronto General Hospital, 21 June 1922 and 7 Oct. 1922.

16. Sir Frederick Banting, Unpublished Manuscript, Banting Papers, Fisher Library, University of Toronto, courtesty Michael Bliss.

17. Ibid., 64-5.

18. Ibid., 65.

19. Bliss, "Banting", op. cit., 307.

CHAPTER X: *The Department Grows and Evolves*

1. Duncan Graham, Letter to Sir Robert Falconer, 8 Sept. 1919. Archives, University of Toronto.
2. Duncan Graham, "Medical Education," *Nova Scotia Medical Bulletin*, 1954, 35:402-14.
3. Norman Wrong, Oral History Tape, Hannah Institute for the History of Medicine.
4. J.D. Hamilton, Oral History Tape.
5. J. Allan Walters, Oral History Tape.
6. Albin T. Jousse, Oral History Tape.
7. Irwin Hilliard, Oral History Tape.
8. Calendar, University of Toronto, 1922-23, Report of Dean Alexander Primrose, Archives, University of Toronto.
9. Henry A. Christian, Letter to Duncan Graham, 8 Nov. 1925, Archives, University of Toronto.
10. University of Toronto Archives, Board of Governors, 12 May 1932, A 70-0024/023, 178.
11. Mark Irish, Chairman's Report, Minutes of Board of Trustees Annual Meeting, 23 Jan. 1935, Archives, Toronto General Hospital.
12. Ibid., 29 Jan. 1936.
13. See Appendix C.
14. University of Toronto Archives, President's Reports, 1919-20, 1938-39.
15. Appendix B, Bibliography of Duncan Graham.

CHAPTER XI: *Marriage and Family*

1. Mrs. L.N. (Mary) Hogarth, Mrs. W.J. (Lorraine) Hovey Sutherland and Dr. Alan Bruce-Robertson, Personal communication to authors.
2. Minutes, Medical Advisory Board, Toronto General Hospital, 8 Nov. 1920 and 6 Dec. 1920.
3. Kathleen McMurrich, Personal communication to RBK.

CHAPTER XII: *Duncan Graham and the Royal College*

1. D. Sclater Lewis, *The Royal College of Physicians and Surgeons of Canada: 1920-1960*, ch. II-IV.
2. Ibid., ch. V.
3. Ibid., 22.
4. Ibid., 25-8.
5. Ibid., 70.
6. Ibid., 144-5; Robert B. Kerr, *History of the Medical Council of Canada* (Medical Council of Canada, 1979), 35.
7. Lewis, op. cit., 141-53, and Kerr, op. cit., 34-7.
8. Lewis, op. cit., 149.
9. Ibid., 196.
10. James H. Graham, personal communication to DW.
11. Minutes, Meeting of Council, Royal College of Physicians and Surgeons of Canada, 1 Nov. 1935.

CHAPTER XIII: *World War II and the Professor's many Hats*

1. Lewis, op. cit., 213. MacDermot, H.E., *One Hundred Years of Medicine in Canada* (Toronto: McClelland and Stewart, 1967), 214-5.

2. Duncan Graham, Letter to Col. R. M. Gorssline, D.G.M.S., R.C.A.M.C., 17 Jan. 1940, Files, Surgeon General of Canada.
3. Annual Reports, Department of Medicine, Archives, University of Toronto.
4. Citation on the Occasion of the Presentation of the Sesquicentennial Long Service Award to Miss Stella Clutton, 1961, Archives, University of Toronto.
5. Minutes, Sub-Executive Committee, Canadian Medical Association, 4 Sept. 1940, 42-3.
6. Minutes, Executive Committee, Canadian Medical Association, 14-15 March 1941, 124.
7. Ibid., 20-21 June 1941, 224-5.
8. Duncan Graham, "Valedictory Address of the President of the Canadian Medical Association", *Can. Med. Assoc. J.*, 1941, 45:177-80.
9. Ibid.
10. Records, Medical Research Council, Courtesy, Dorothy J. Wright, Secretary of Council.

CHAPTER XIV: *Easing Up*

1. Citations: D.Sc., University of Western Ontario, LL.D., University of Toronto, LL.D., Queen's University, Archives, University of Toronto.
2. John D. Hamilton, "The First Sir John and Lady Eaton Professor of Medicine," read before the Medical Historical Club, Toronto, October 1978; Personal Communication to RBK.
3. Duncan Graham, personal communication with RBK.
4. Robert B. Kerr, personal recollections.
5. Ibid.
6. Alan Bruce-Robertson, Personal Communication to DW.
7. Gordon Fahrni, Personal Communication to RBK.
8. Duncan Graham, Letter to RBK, 21 Aug. 1969.
9. Mrs. L. N. Hogarth (Enid Mary), Personal Communication to RBK.

EPILOGUE

1. *Toronto Daily Star*, 13 June 1947, 4.

APPENDICES

APPENDIX A

THE SIR JOHN AND LADY EATON FELLOWSHIP

Reproduced below is the original agreement between Sir John and Lady Eaton and the University of Toronto. Subsequent agreements have been made to ensure the continuing association and benefaction.

THIS INDENTURE made in duplicate this Ninth day of January in the year of our Lord, one thousand nine hundred and nineteen.

BETWEEN:—

SIR JOHN C. EATON, Knight, and *FLORA MCRAE LADY EATON*, and *THE T. EATON CO. LIMITED* of the City of Toronto, hereinafter called the "donors" where the context so permits,
OF THE FIRST PART;
—and—
THE GOVERNORS OF THE UNIVERSITY OF TORONTO, hereinafter called the "Governors"
OF THE SECOND PART;

W H E R E A S there is now established in connection with the Faculty of Medicine at the University of Toronto, a Department of General Medicine as an integral part of the educational system of the University, and there is now applied and expended out of the general income of the University in connection with such Department the annual sum of thirteen thousand dollars ($13,000.00) or thereabouts.

AND WHEREAS the Donors propose, upon the terms and conditions hereinafter mentioned, to provide an annual income which shall, with the annual sum above referred to, be expended in connection with the said Department and the maintenance thereof and the Governors agree to accept the same on the terms and conditions hereinafter expressed.

NOW THEREFORE THIS INDENTURE WITNESSETH that the parties agree as follows:—

1. The Donor, The T. Eaton Co. Limited will pay to the Governors the sum of five hundred thousand dollars ($500,000.00) in twenty equal annual payments of twenty-five thousand ($25,000.00) each on the Ninth day of January in each year, the first payment to be made on the Ninth day of January, 1919, and the last of such payments to be made on the Ninth day of January, 1938. The payments so made shall be known as the "EATON ENDOWMENT".

2. The Governors agree to set aside in each year of the twenty years during which the above payments are to be made for the purpose of the said Department and for expenditure in connnection therewith a sum which in any event shall not be less that thirteen thousand ($13,000.00) dollars per year.

3. The annual sum of twenty-five thousand dollars ($25,000.00), and the said annual sum to be set aside under paragraph 2 hereof, (the whole of which are hereinafter sometimes referred to as the "Income") shall be expended yearly in connection with the Department of General Medicine on the recommendation of the President with whom shall act in an advisory capacity the Committee, hereinafter referred to and upon the abolition of the Committee, in lieu thereof, the Head of the Department of General Medicine.

4. A Committee shall be appointed by the Governors on the recommendation of the President of the university, which Committee shall always include the Donors Sir John C. Eaton and Lady Eaton and a representative named by the same donors and two members of the Medical profession named by the said Donors.

5. In the event of any vacancies in the Committee, the President after consultation with the Donors shall recommend a name or names to the Governors and the vacancies shall be filled by the Governors on such recommendation.

6. The Committee shall continue in existence until the payments herein provided for are fully paid or until an unanimous recommendation of the President, the Dean of the Faculty of Medicine, the Permanent Head of the Department of Medicine to be appointed and the Donors Sir John C. Eaton and Lady Eaton recommending the abolition of the Committee is presented to the Governors.

7. The Committee shall act generally in an advisory capacity with the President in connection with the re-organization of the Department of General Medicine and with the President and Permanent Head of the Department in connection with the direction of and policy of the Department after re-organization thereof and without limiting the above.

(a) In an advisory capacity with the president in connection with the appointing of the Permanent Head of the Department the whole of whose time shall be given to the Department and also the remuneration of such Permanent Head.

(b) In an advisory capacity with the President and the Permanent Head of the Department with regard to the expenditure of the "income" in connection with the Department, and especially, with regard to the apportionment of the "income" between the sub-departments including the apportionment with regard to the sub-department of Pediatrics.

(c) As to the time when the sub-department of Pediatrics shall be specially developed as hereinafter mentioned and the portion of the said "income" to be thereafter expended in connection with such sub-department.

8. It is the desire of the donors that when a proper time has arrived the sub-department of Pediatrics should be emphasized and specially developed, under the Head of the Department of General Medicine and that the Head of such sub-department of Pediatrics should be required to give at least half of his time to such sub-department.

9. The Head of the Department of General Medicine shall recommend to the President for appointment and dismissal all men in his Department whether under salary and giving their whole time to the work in which they are engaged or whether receiving an honorarium and giving part only of their time or whether giving their time without honorarium or salary.

10. Upon failure at any time of the Governors to carry out the terms of this agreement and especially the second paragraph hereof all obligations hereunder on the part of the Donors shall cease and determine.

11. The Donors Sir John C. Eaton and Lady Eaton shall not be liable in respect of any of the payments or obligations undertaken by the Donors hereunder but the Donor The T. Eaton Co. Limited shall be solely liable therefor, such liability being accepted by the Governors to the exclusion of any liability on the part of the other Donors.

THIS AGREEMENT shall extend to any be binding upon the heir, executors, administrators, successors and assigns of the respective parties hereto.

IN WITNESS WHEREOF Sir John C. Eaton and Flora McCrae Lady Eaton have hereunderto set their hands and seals and the T. Eaton Co. Limited has caused its Corporate Seal to be affixed under the hands of its proper officers in that behalf, and the said Party of the Second Part has caused its Corporate Seal to be affixed under the hands of its proper officers in that behalf.

SIGNED, SEALED AND DELIVERED,

in the presence of

APPENDIX B

PUBLICATIONS OF DUNCAN GRAHAM

Graham, D. Leucocytes and leucocytosis. Dominion Med. Monthly, Toronto 28: 145-153, 1907.

Nasmith, G.G., and Graham, D.A.L. The haematology of carbon monoxide poisoning. J. Physiol. 35: 32-52, 1907.

White, W.C., and Graham, D.A.L. On the increased infective power produced in bacteria by sensitization with normal serum of the same species. J. Med. Res. 20: 67-78, 1909.

White, W.C., and Graham, D.A.L. A quantitative modification of the Von Pirquet tuberculin reaction and its value in diagnosis and prognosis. J. Med. Res. 20: 347-357, 1909.

White, W.C., and Graham, D.A.L. Studies on the action of sera on tuberculin cutaneous reaction. J.Med. Res. 21: 261-265, 1909.

White, W.C., and Graham, D.A.L., and Van Norman, K.H., An index to tuberculin treatment in tuberculosis by the minimal cutaneous reaction method. J. Med. Res. 21: 255-260, 1909. [also Trans. Assoc. Amer. Phys. 24: 129-134, 1909].

White, W.C., Graham, D.A.L. , and Van Norman, K.H. Studies of tuberculin reaction, with a new index to dosage in tuberculin treatment. Trans. Fifth Annual Meeting of the National Association for the Study and Prevention of Tuberculosis. 1909, 223-228.

Gräfe, E., und Graham, D.A.L. Luxus-Konsumption Deutsches Kongress für Innerer Medizin, Wiesbaden, 1911.

Gräfe, E., und Graham, D.A.L. Über die Anpassungsfähigkeit des tierischen Organismus an überreichliche Nahrungszufuhr (Nach Versuchen am Hunde). Hoppe-Seyler's Ztschr. f. Physiol. Chem. 73: 1-67, 1911.

Gräfe, E., und Graham, D.A.L. Untersuchugen über Isolyse. Münch. Med. Wochenschr. 43: 2257-2260, 1911.

Kraus, R., Graham, D.A.L., und Zia, Z. Über Hämatoxine und die Blutplatten-methode. Deutsche Med. Wochenschr. 32: 1471-1473, 1911.

Graham, D. Epidemiology of anterior poliomyelitis. Canad. J. Med. Surg. 37: 57-61, 1915.

Oille, J.A., Graham, D., and Detweiler, H.K. Streptococcus bacteremia in endo-carditis; its presence before and after the development of endocardial signs. Trans. Assoc. Amer. Phys. **30**: 674-697, 1915.

Graham, D. Some points in the diagnosis and treatment of dysentery occuring in the British Salonika Force. Lancet **1**: 51-55, 1918.

Graham, D. Clinical aspects of bacillary dysentery. Nelson Loose Leaf Medicine **2**: 177, 1923.

Graham, D. Diabetes mellitus and insulin. Univ. Toronto Med. Bull. April, 1923.

Graham, D. Pleural infections. Canad. Med. Assoc. J. **13**: 863-865, 1923.

Oille, J.A., Graham, D., and Detweiler, H.K. A further report on a series of recov-ered cases of subacute bacterial endocarditis. Trans. Assoc. Amer. Phys. **39**: 227-230, 1924.

Graham, D. The use and abuse of iodine in the treatment of goitre. Canad. Med. Assoc. J. **14**: 821-823, 1924.

Graham, D. The treatment of acidosis and coma in diabetes mellitus. Med. J. Austral. **2**: 78-80, 1925. [also Tran. Amer. Ther. Soc., 1924]

Graham, D. The aetiology of anaemia and its importance in diagnosis and treatment. Univ. Toronto Med. Bull. March 1926. [also Proc. Inter-State Postgraduate Med. Assembly of Amer. 1925]

Graham, D. Addison's (pernicious) anaemia. Canad. Med. Assoc. J. **16**: 881-886, 1926.

Graham, D. Aetiology and clinical manifestations of anaemia. Canad. Med. Assoc. J. **17**: 393-396, 1927.

Graham D., Farquharson, R.F., and Maltby, E.J. Observations on the size of the red blood corpuscles before and after splenectomy in haemolytic jaundice. J. Clin. Invest. **4**: 452-453, 1927 (abstract).

Graham, D. The treatment of pernicious anaemia. Canad. Med. Assoc. J. **19**: 150-153, 1928.

Hepburn, J., and Graham, D. An electrocardiographic study on 123 cases of diabetes mellitus. Trans. Assoc. Amer. Phys. **43**: 86-94, 1928. [also Amer. J. Med. Sci. **176**: 782-789, 1928].

Graham, D., Focal infection. Oral Health **3**: 138-141, 1928.

Graham, D. The teaching of physical diagnosis. Bull. Assoc. Amer. Coll. **3**: 115-119, 1928.

Graham, D., Farquharson, R.F., Borsook, H., and Goulding, A.M. Urobilinogen excretion in Addison's "pernicious" anaemia before and after liver therapy. J. Clin Invest. **7**: 510-511, 1929 (abstract).

Graham, D. Subacute and chronic nephritis. Canad. Med. Assoc. J. **20**: 144-145, 1929.

Graham, D. The differential diagnosis of clinical conditions accompanied by jaundice. Canad. Med. Assoc. J. **21**: 380-383, 1929. [also Univ. Toronto Med. J. **7**: 34-38, 1929].

Graham, D. The differential diagnosis of superficial glandular swellings. Canad. Med. Assoc. J. **22**: 324-326, 1930.

Fraquharson, R.F., and Graham, D. Liver therapy in the treatment of subacute combined degeneration of the cord. Canad. med. Assoc. J. **23**: 237-244, 1930.

Graham, D., and Fletcher, A.A. The large bowel in chronic arthritis. Amer. J. Med. Sci. **179**: 91-93, 1930. [also Trans. Assoc. Amer. Phys. **44**: 231-237, 1929].

Graham, D. Focal infection. Canad. Med. Assoc. J. **25**: 422-424, 1931.

Farquharson, R.F., and Graham, D. Cases of Simmonds' disease. Trans. Assoc. Amer. Phys. **46**: 150-161, 1931.

Warner, W.P., and Graham, D. Lobar atelectasis as a cause of triangular roentgen shadows in bronchiectasis. Arch. Int. Med. **52**: 888-904, 1933.

Graham, D. Chronic arterial occlusion of the extremities. Ann. Int. Med. **7**: 431-438, 1933.

Graham, D. The clinical diagnosis of arteriosclerosis and hypertension. Canad. Med. Assoc. J. **32**: 29-34, 1935.

Graham, D. the diagnosis of hepatic disorders. Canad. Med. Assoc. J. **33**: 247-250, 1935.

Graham, D. Undergraduate instruction in medicine. J. Assoc. Amer. Med. Coll. **11**: 213-218, 1936.

Graham, D. Embolism and thrombosis of the larger arteries: their diagnosis and treatment. Canad. Med. Assoc. J. **36**: 33-38, 1937.

Graham, D. Diseases of the Blood Vessels. Oxford Loose Leaf System of Medicine. New York: Oxford University Press, 1937. Vol. 2; Chap. 14.

Graham, D., and Hyland, H.H. Observations on the treatment of respiratory paralysis in adult poliomyelitis. Trans. Assoc. Amer. Phys. **53**: 165-171, 1938.

Rykert, H.E., and Graham, D. Some problems in the diagnosis, prognosis and treatment of acute arterial occlusions. Amer. Heart J. **15**: 395-401, 1938.

Graham, D., Warner, W.P., Dauphinee, J.A., and Dickson, R.C. The treatment of pneumococcal pneumonia with Dagenan (M & B 693). Canad. Med. Assoc. J. **40**: 325-332, 1939.

Graham, D., Warner, W.P., Dauphinee, J.A., and Dickson, R.C. The treatment of 100 cases of pneumococcal pneumonia with Dagenan (sulfapyridine). Trans. Assoc. Amer. Phys. **54**: 98-111, 1939.

Graham, D. Erythraemia — polycythaemia rubra vera. Canad. Med. Assoc. J. **42**: 281-284, 1940.

Graham, D. Valedictory address of the President of the Canadian Medical Association. Canad. Med. Assoc. J. **45**: 177-180, 1941.

Graham, D. Medical education. Nova Scotia Med. Bull. **35**: 402-414, 1956.

APPENDIX C

RESIDENT PHYSICIANS IN THE DEPARTMENT OF MEDICINE, TORONTO GENERAL HOSPITAL AND FELLOWS IN THE DEPARTMENT OF MEDICINE, UNIVERSITY OF TORONTO, 1923-1947

1923-24	Dr. William P. Warner
1924-25	Dr. William P. Warner (resigned because of illness) replaced by Dr. R.S. Lang
1925-26	Dr. Ray F. Farquharson
1926-27	Dr. Ray F. Farquharson
1927-28	Dr. Ernest J. Maltby
1928-29	Dr. Ernest J. Maltby
1929-30	Dr. William J. Gardiner
1930-31	Dr. William J. Gardiner
1931-32	Dr. W. Hurst Brown
1932-33	Dr. Edward A. Keenleyside

1933-34	Dr. George C. Ferguson
1934-35	Dr. George C. Ferguson
1935-36	Dr. Arthur E. Parkes
1936-37	Dr. Robert B. Kerr
1937-38	Dr. Fred C. Heal
1938-39	Dr. Robert C. Dickson
1939-40	Dr. William A. Ollie
1940-41	Dr. Arthur W. Bagnall
1941-42	Dr. Keith J.R. Wightman
1942-43	Dr. Herbert B. Wallis
1943-44	Dr. Allan J. Longmore
1944-45	Dr. R. Lancey Stirrett
1945-46	Dr. William F. Greenwood
1946-47	Dr. D.B. Kelly

APPENDIX D

PHYSICIANS WHO RECEIVED TRAINING UNDER DUNCAN GRAHAM IN ADDITION TO THOSE WHO WERE RESIDENTS IN THE DEPARTMENT OF MEDICINE

Dr. M. Alexander
Dr. C.W.J. Armstrong
Dr. W.B. Arnup
Dr. G.R. Balfour
Dr. H.J.M. Barnett
Dr. J.R. Bingham
Dr. E.S. Bird
Dr. E.C. Blackhall
Dr. F.S. Brien
Dr. E.F. Brooks
Dr. E. Broughton
Dr. C.B. Brown
Dr. K.W.G. Brown
Dr. H.A. Burnett
Dr. C.R. Burton
Dr. W.B. Charles
Dr. W.T.W. Clarke
Dr. M.F. Clarkson
Dr. A.C. Coatsworth
Dr. J.E.C. Cole
Dr. W.F. Connell
Dr. T.A. Crowther
Dr. B.P. Danard
Dr. J.A. Dauphinee
Dr. Jean Davey
Dr. H.D. Delamere
Dr. A. Douglas

Dr. J.G. Falconer
Dr. F.W. Farley
Dr. K.E. Ferrie
Dr. G.W. Fitzgerald
Dr. J.L. Fowler
Dr. R.R. Gerred
Dr. J.W. Gibson
Dr. A.F. Graham
Dr. D.C. Graham
Dr. J.W. Graham
Dr. C.C. Gray
Dr. H.M. Gray
Dr. H.C. Hair
Dr. W.E. Hall
Dr. G.P. Hamblin
Dr. W.A. Hawke
Dr. J.A. Hildes
Dr. I.M. Hilliard
Dr. F.W.B. Hurlburt
Dr. H.H. Hyland
Dr. C.H. Jaimet
Dr. E.S. Jeffrey
Dr. A.M. Johnston
Dr. MacA. Johnston
Dr. J.E. Josephson
Dr. A.T. Jousse
Dr. H.G. Kelly

Dr. A.J. Kerwin
Dr. C. Krikpatrick
Dr. M.O. Klotz
Dr. J.A. Laidlaw
Dr. A.M. Large
Dr. G. Lea
Dr. G.A. Low
Dr. R.I. Macdonald
Dr. D.J. MacKenzie
Dr. R.W. McBain
Dr. J.F. McCreary
Dr. J.C. McGarry
Dr. J.A. McGeachy
Dr. N.B. McGillivray
Dr. D.L. McIntosh
Dr. A.D. McKelvey
Dr. J.A. Mclren
Dr. N.R. McMurchy
Dr. W.A. McTavish
Dr. J.W. Magladery
Dr. G.W. Manners
Dr. G.W. Manning
Dr. J.D. Markham
Dr. J.A.D. Marquis
Dr. J. Meiners
Dr. A. Montgomery
Dr. J. Mongomery

Dr. D. Murnaghan	Dr. W.I. Sparks	Dr. J.A. Walters
Dr. F.L. Nichols	Dr. R.L. Stirritt	Dr. J.G. Watt
Dr. M.A. Ogryzlo	Dr. N.C. Slade	Dr. W.K. Welsh
Dr. W.E. Pugsley	Dr. A.H. Squires	Dr. G. Whillans
Dr. J. Rathbun	Dr. K. Swallow	Dr. R.W. Will
Dr. J.G. Reid	Dr. R. M. Taylor	Dr. A.R. Wilkins
Dr. J.C. Richardson	Dr. J.A. Traynor	Dr. G.E. Wodehouse
Dr. J.W. Scott	Dr. E.J. Trow	Dr. M.A. Woodside
Dr. H.A. Simms	Dr. F.A. Turnbull	Dr. H.A. Wrong
Dr. J.C. Sinclair	Dr. H.B. Wallis	Dr. N.M. Wrong

APPENDIX E

DUNCAN GRAHAM AWARD RECIPIENTS

1969	Dr. John P. Hubbard	1981	Dr. Donald R. Wilson
1971	Dr. Walter C. Mackenzie	1982	Dr. Angus D. McLachlin
1972	Dr. Douglas E. Cannell	1983	Dr. Ronald V. Christie
1974	Dr. Robert C. Dickson	1984	Dr. Martin M. Hoffman
1975	Dr. William Boyd		(posthumous)
1976	Dr. Eugene Robillard	1985	Dr. Fraser N. Gurd
1977	Dr. John F. McCreary	1986	Dr. Charles P. Leblond
1978	Dr. Lea C. Steeves	1987	Dr. Hugh Allen
1979	Dr. J.S.L. Browne	1988	Dr. Pierre Bois
1980	Dr. J. Wendell MacLeod		

APPENDIX F

1. Members of the Department of Medicine, University of Toronto as Listed in the Calendar of 1918-1919 (Before Appointment of Duncan Graham)

Professor of Medicine and Clinical Medicine — Alexander McPhedran
Associate Professor of Medicine and Clinical Medicine — J.T. Fotheringham
Associate Professors of Clinical Medicine — Allen M. Baines (Paediatrics), W.B. Thistle, R.J. Dwyer, H.B. Anderson, Graham Chambers, William Goldie, John Ferguson.
Associates in Clinical Medicine — H.C. Parsons, W.J. McCallum, J.H. Elliott, G.W. Howland, H.S. Hutchison.
Demonstrators in Clinical Medicine — E.C. Burson, F.A. Clarkson, B. O'Reilly, D. King Smith, C.J. Wagner, J.H. McPhedran, C.S. McVicar, G.S. Strathy, W.F. McPhedran, G.W. Ross, R.W. Mann, G.H. Young, A.J. MacKenzie.
Assistants in Clinical Medicine — J.A. Oille, J.D. Loudon, G.F. Boyer, M.B. White, T.J. Page, G. Bates, F.S. Park, R.G. Armour, F.S. Minns, E.J. Trow, C. Sheard Jr., T.J. Glover.
Professor of Therapeutics — R.D. Rudolf.

2. Members of the Department of Medicine, University of Toronto as Listed in the Calendar of 1920-21 (After Appointment of Duncan Graham)

Emeritus Professor of Medicine — Alexander McPhedran.
Professor of Medicine — Duncan Graham
Associate Professor of Medicine — William Goldie.
Clinicians in Medicine — R.G. Armour, G.F. Boyer, W.R. Campbell, A.H. Caulfied, F.A. Clarkson, H.K. Detweiler, J.H. Elliott, A.A. Fletcher, N. Gwyn, G.W. Howland, H.S. Hutchison, R. Jamieson, N.M. Keith, J.D. Loudon, D. McGillivray, A.C. McPhedran, J.H. McPhedran, W.F. McPhedran, A.J. MacKenzie, F.S. Minns, L. Murray, W. Ogden, J.A. Oille, T.J. Page, H.C. Parson, F.W. Rolph, D. King Smith, Charles Sheard Jr., G.S. Strathy, E.J. Trow, M.B. White, G.S. Young.

LIST OF ILLUSTRATIONS

All illustrations are from the family collection except the picture of the lacrosse team, which is reproduced courtesy the University of Toronto Archives, and the pictures of Sir John and Lady Eaton, which are reproduced courtesy the T. Eaton Co. Archives.

INDEX